CARDIOMYOPATHIES

ACQUIRED CONDITIONS PRIMARILY AFFECTING PRESSURE/VOLUME LOAD

THE AGEING HEART

Provided as a service to medicine by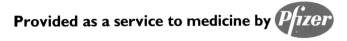

Produced and published by Gower Medical Publishing, London.

Robert H Anderson BSc, MD, FRCPath

Joseph Levy Professor of Paediatric Cardiac Morphology

National Heart and Lung Institute

Royal Brompton National Heart and Lung Hospital

London, UK

Anton E Becker MD

Professor of Pathology

Head, Department of Cardiovascular Pathology

Academic Medical Centre

University of Amsterdam

The Netherlands

Selected chapters reprinted from *The Heart: Structure in Health and Disease* by Robert H Anderson and Anton E Becker

The sponsorship of this book does not imply approval or otherwise
of any of the products of the sponsor by the authors or editors.

Printed in Singapore by Imago Productions (FE) Pte Ltd.

CARDIOMYOPATHIES

Initially, the term cardiomyopathy was applied to any disorder affecting heart muscle. In 1980, a task force of the World Health Organisation and the International Society of Federations of Cardiology suggested that a distinction should be made between disorders of myocardium having a known cause or those associated with systemic disease, and those with an unknown cause. The former were grouped together as 'specific heart-muscle diseases'. Thus, conditions such as glycogen storage disease and amyloidosis fall in the group of specific diseases (see above). The latter group has been termed 'cardiomyopathy'. A division has since been made: this includes dilated cardiomyopathy, hypertrophic cardiomyopathy, and restrictive cardiomyopathy. Since then, however, it has become apparent that this categorization in itself is less than perfect. In some instances, it may prove impossible, clinically, to distinguish between the restrictive and dilated types. In other cases, the pathology encountered in a 'typical' case of restrictive cardiomyopathy may not fit with the 'classical' concept (see below). Furthermore, the terminology chosen suggests that hypertrophy occurs only in hypertrophic cardiomyopathy, which is definitely not the case. So-called arrhythmogenic right ventricular dysplasia is also a disorder of unknown cause and, hence, should be included within the category of cardiomyopathies. The condition is discussed in this section.

Dilated cardiomyopathy

Dilated cardiomyopathy can occur at almost any age and is characterized by symptoms and signs of congestive heart failure, often rapidly progressive. Disturbances of rhythm may be a serious complication. From a pathophysiologic point of view, the disease is characterized by decreased myocardial contractility. The diagnosis is based on the exclusion of all other forms of congestive cardiomyopathies. This may pose a problem since other diseases, such as alcoholic cardiomyopathy and the vast majority of cases of myocarditis, are not readily diagnosed. Endomyocardial biopsies may be helpful (see Chapter 10).

A particular form of dilated cardiomyopathy is associated with pregnancy and is known also as postpartum (or peripartum) cardiomyopathy.

In dilated cardiomyopathy, the heart is enlarged with dilatation of all four chambers (Fig. 12.1). Such dilatation may mask the presence of hypertrophy. The gross aspect of the myocardium is usually unremarkable, and the endocardium almost always shows diffuse or patchy fibroelastosis (Fig. 12.2). Intracavitary thrombosis is common both macro- and microscopically.

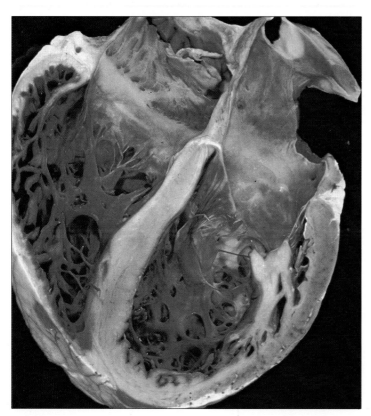

Fig. 12.1   Four-chamber section in dilated cardiomyopathy showing dilatation of both ventricles with marked wall-thinning.

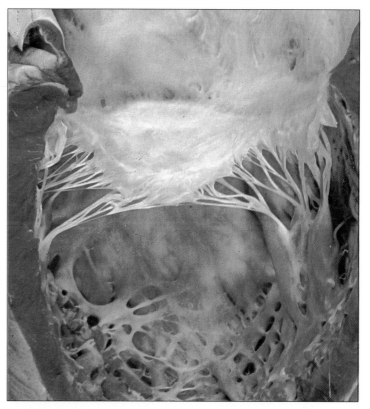

Fig. 12.2   Extensive endocardial fibroelastosis of left ventricle in dilated cardiomyopathy.

The histopathological features of the myocardium are nonspecific. Endomyocardial biopsies will reveal distinct hypertrophy of myocytes (Fig. 12.3) with a varying degree of interstitial fibrosis. Occasionally, particularly in patients in whom the lapse between the onset of symptoms and the biopsy is less than six months, scant inflammatory cells, usually lymphocytes and macrophages, may be seen (Fig. 12.4). Sometimes, the endocardium present in the biopsy specimens may reveal thickening by fibroelastic tissue and the presence of smooth-muscle cells (Fig. 12.5). These observations of the myocardium in patients with dilated cardiomyopathy are often in striking contrast with the pathology seen at autopsy. In the latter instance, the myocardial cells are often excessively attenuated.

Lymphocytes may often be present in biopsy samples of the myocardium in patients with dilated cardiomyopathy. This fact, coupled with the observations made in patients affected by viral myocarditis, some of whom may develop the clinical picture of dilated cardiomyopathy without identifiable traces of a previous viral infection, have led to the assumption that, at least in some patients, dilated cardiomyopathy may be an end stage of a viral myocarditis. This is further strengthened by *in situ* hybridization of endomyocardial biopsies of patients with dilated cardiomyopathy, which occasionally demonstrate the presence of RNA sequences of Coxsackie B viruses.

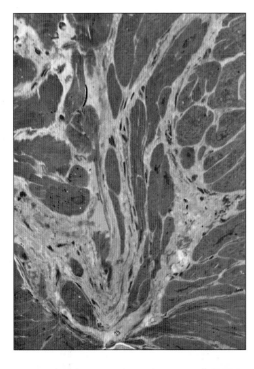

Fig. 12.3 Endomyocardial biopsy. Distinct hypertrophy of myocytes with interstitial fibrosis. (Toluidine blue stain.)

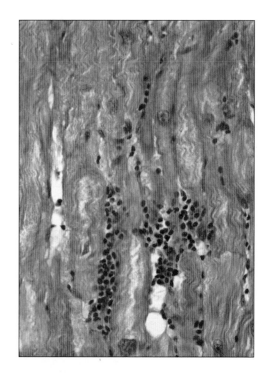

Fig. 12.4 Endomyocardial biopsy in dilated cardiomyopathy. Amidst hypertrophic myocytes scant lymphocytic infiltrates are present. (H&E stain.)

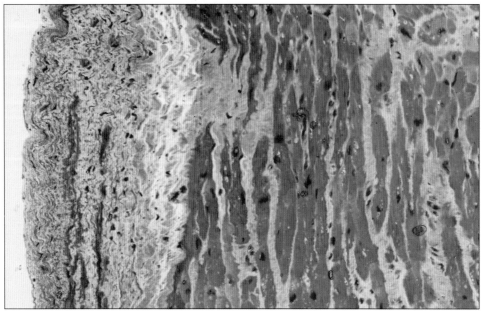

Fig. 12.5 Endomyocardial biopsy in dilated cardiomyopathy. Endocardial thickening contains smooth muscle cells. (Toluidine blue stain.)

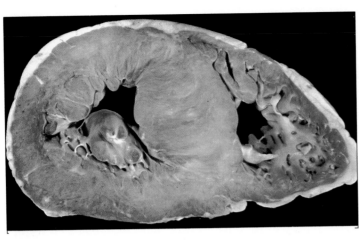

Fig. 12.6 Transverse section in hypertrophic cardiomyopathy shows asymmetric septal hypertrophy.

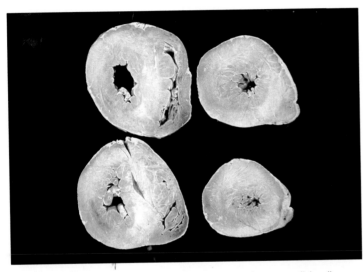

Fig. 12.7 Hypertrophic cardiomyopathy: asymmetric myocardial wall thickening extends from ventricular septum into anterior wall with almost circumferential spread in apical region. Note marked fibrosis (whitish area).

Hypertrophic cardiomyopathy

The clinical presentation of the hypertrophic form varies considerably and includes angina pectoris, syncope, cardiac failure, and sudden death. Some patients may be totally asymptomatic. The basic pathophysiologic abnormality is a decrease in diastolic myocardial distensibility.

The 'classical' pathologic feature is asymmetrical hypertrophy of the ventricular septum (Fig. 12.6). This condition should be distinguished from 'disproportionate ventricular septal thickening'. The latter may occur as a nonspecific condition in various types of congenital heart malformations, in aortic valvar stenosis, or in the adaptive left ventricular hypertrophy observed in the heart of athletes.

Many hearts with unequivocal hypertrophic cardiomyopathy do not present the classical features as outlined above. Indeed, some cases may present symmetric hypertrophy, while others may show asymmetric hypertrophy involving other areas of the left ventricle and the septum, particularly the apical region (Fig.12.7).

Even in cases with 'classical' asymmetric hypertrophy, the ventricular abnormality usually extends into the anterior left ventricular free wall. In case of septal asymmetry, the left ventricular endocardial surface shows a fibrous thickening, almost like an imprint of the overlying aortic leaflet of the mitral valve, most likely due to the impact of the leaflet during diastole (Fig. 12.8). The mere observation of this endocardial thickening on the septum may suggest the presence of hypertrophic cardiomyopathy. This may then be significant in evaluating the cause of death in young individuals dying in a sudden and unexpected fashion.

The cut surface of the abnormal thickened areas of myocardium often reveals an unusual texture of the myocardium, frequently accompanied by fibrosis (Fig. 12.9). The histological appearance of the areas of myocardium affected grossly in this fashion is that of a marked disorganization of the myofibrils

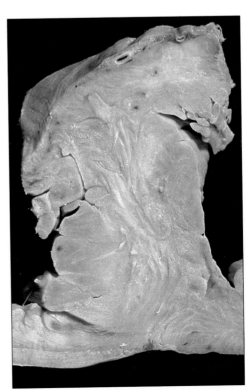

Fig. 12.9 Transverse section through ventricular septum in hypertrophic cardiomyopathy shows bizarre fibre arrangement.

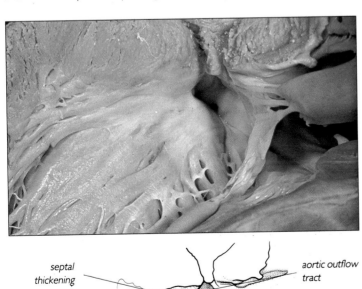

septal thickening

aortic outflow tract

endocardial thickening

mitral valve

Fig. 12.8 Hypertrophic cardiomyopathy showing narrowed left ventricular outflow tract and endocardial thickening of septum.

(Fig. 12.10). The abnormally short and broad muscle fibres often run in different directions, showing complex bridging of adjacent fibres with abnormal intercellular contacts, leading to the formation of whirls. The myocytes are distinctly hypertrophic, with hyperchromatic and often bizarre nuclei (Fig. 12.11). The diameter of the individual myocytes often measures 90–100µm, as compared with the range of 5–12µm in normal hearts and an average diameter of cells hypertrophied due to any other cause of approximately 20–25µm.

An increased cellular branching and extensive side-to-side intercellular junctions are also noted ultrastructurally (Fig. 12.12).

In themselves, neither the light-microscopic nor the ultrastructural changes are unique for hypertrophic cardiomyopathy. Nevertheless, the gross appearance, together with the extent of the microscopic changes will lead almost without exception to a proper diagnosis of this condition. It is important to realize, however, that 'disorganization' as such, particularly when observed in small samples, is not diagnostic for hypertrophic cardiomyopathy. This is particularly the case when evaluating endomyocardial biopsies. Naturally occurring 'disorganization' is common subendocardially on both the right and left sides of the ventricular septum.

The deranged architecture of myocardial fibres in hypertrophic cardiomyopathy is often further complicated by excessive fibrosis (Fig. 12.13) and, occasionally, by myocardial infarction. Such fibrotic changes are usually accompanied by extensive obstructive changes in intramural coronary arteries, characterized by a proliferation of longitudinally orientated smooth-muscle cells within the intimal layer (Fig. 12.14).

The aetiology and pathogenesis of hypertrophic cardiomyopathy remain as yet unknown. An autosomal dominant pattern of inheritance has now been established in familial cases and it has been shown that, in this kindred, the gene responsible is located on chromosome 14.

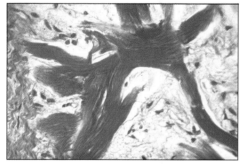

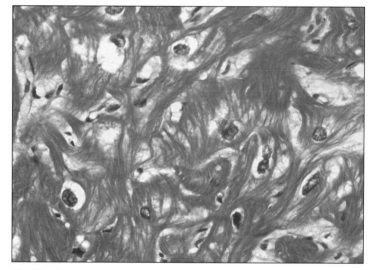

Fig. 12.10 Histology of hypertrophic cardiomyopathy: (upper) disarray in infant heart; (lower) high power bizarre| perpendicular branching amidst fibrosis. E-VG (upper), Mallory's trichrome stain (lower).

Fig. 12.11 Histological section of young adult heart in hypertrophic cardiomyopathy shows combination of unusual texture with excessive hypertrophy and intracellular abnormalities. H&E stain.

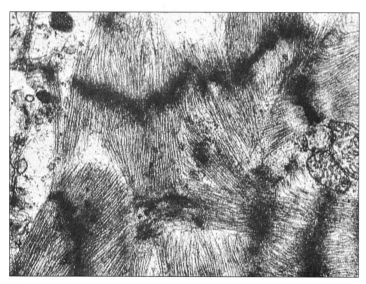

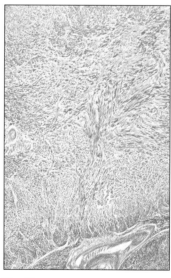

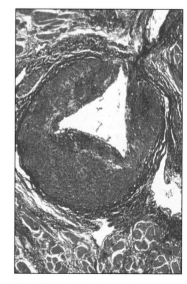

Fig. 12.12 Ultrastructural appearances of hypertrophic cardiomyopathy include disorientated myofibrils, interweaving myofilaments and irregular Z-bands. EM, × 29,400. By courtesy of Dr K.P. Dingemans.

Fig. 12.13 Marked interstitial fibrosis (blue-green). Mallory's trichrome stain.

Fig. 12.14 Histology of hypertrophic cardiomyopathy: intramural coronary artery with hypertrophic media and muscularization leading to luminal narrowing. E-VG stain.

Restrictive cardiomyopathy

This restricted form of cardiomyopathy is characterized functionally by a loss of ventricular compliance. The left ventricle is resistant to filling and demands high diastolic filling pressure. Systolic function is normal.

Cardiac amyloidosis long served as the classical example of restrictive cardiomyopathy. The current definition, however, dictates that amyloidosis is categorized as a 'specific heart-muscle disease'. Nevertheless, this disorder may be one of the most important conditions to be excluded; endomyocardial biopsies may be helpful in this respect. Furthermore, disease characterized primarily by loss of systolic force, such as dilated cardiomyopathy, may eventually be further complicated by loss of compliance, this occurring consequent to myocardial injury and interstitial fibrosis. Thus, dilated cardiomyopathy may eventually turn into a restrictive type of cardiomyopathy. This is yet another example of the deficiencies of the current classification of cardiomyopathy. Indeed, loss of compliance and systolic force may represent extremes of a spectrum of myocardial lesions. Clinical characteristics of both may occur in some patients with end-stage cardiac disease. This has been designated collectively as 'mildly dilated cardiomyopathy'.

Presently, the 'typical' example of restrictive cardiomyopathy is characterized by a heart of normal size but with ventricular cavities that are markedly obliterated by extensive endocardial thickening (Fig. 12.15). The apparatus of the atrioventricular valves is usually included in the obliterative change. Histology reveals endomyocardial fibrosis (Fig. 12.16). These changes probably represent 'end-stage' disease. At earlier stages, the disease may be characterized by an inflammatory process, with an eosinophilic cellular infiltration often accompanied by an early proliferative endocardial reaction (Fig. 12.17). These abnormalities may be revealed in endomyocardial biopsies.

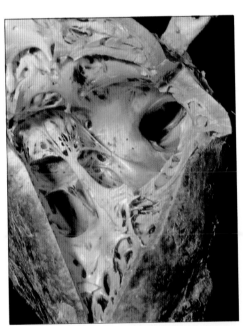

Fig. 12.15 Opened right ventricular outflow tract in a heart with restrictive cardiomyopathy caused by endomyocardial fibrosis. There is endocardial thickening with partial obliteration of the right ventricular apex.

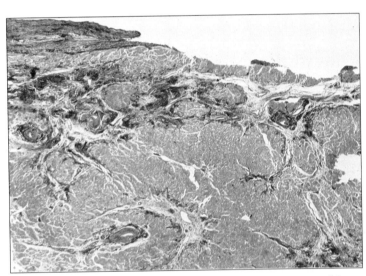

Fig. 12.16 Histological section of left ventricular wall in endomyocardial fibrosis showing fibroelastic thickening of endocardium and fibrosis extending into myocardium. E-VG stain.

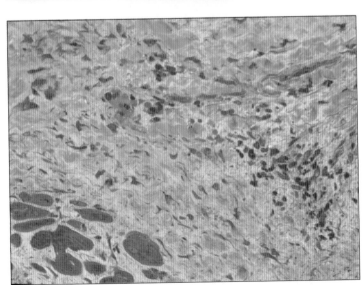

Fig. 12.17 Endomyocardial biopsy in restrictive cardiomyography. There is endomyocardial thickening which contains an inflammatory cellular infiltrate.

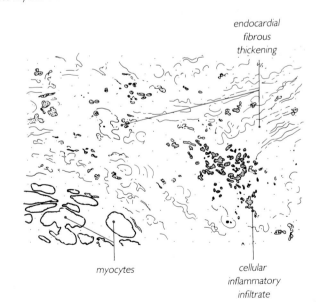

endocardial fibrous thickening

myocytes

cellular inflammatory infiltrate

Apart from this 'classical' histopathological picture, cases do occur with none of these features; instead, the pathology is dominated by extensive interstitial fibrosis (Fig. 12.18). Such examples may reflect end-stage disease of a disorder which, initially, may have presented as heart failure of unknown cause.

Arrhythmogenic right ventricular dysplasia

Arrhythmogenic right ventricular dysplasia is characterized by excessive fatty infiltration of the myocardium, particularly in the right ventricle. Sites of predilection occur in the right ventricular inflow, particularly in its inferior border, in the apex of the right ventricle, and in the anterior wall of the right ventricular infundibulum. The condition is important because of its association with ventricular arrhythmias and sudden death.

The gross appearance of the heart is that of fatty replacement of the myocardium (Fig. 12.19). Microscopical studies will reveal that the myocardium has been extensively replaced by fat (Fig. 12.20). The disease is not restricted to the right ventricle, but may also extend into the left ventricle (Fig. 12.21). The aetiology and pathogenesis of this condition remain as yet unclear (see Fig. 11.1).

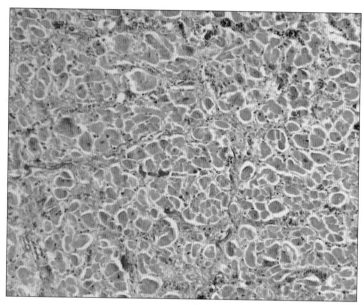

Fig. 12.18 Histological section of myocardium showing extensive interstitial fibrosis. The patient presented the clinical picture of 'restrictive cardiomyopathy'. (EVG stain.)

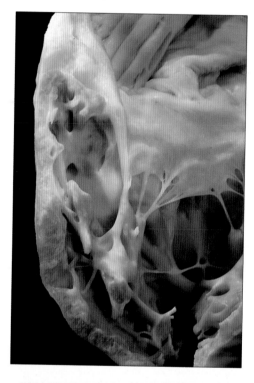

Fig. 12.19 Arrhythmogenic right ventricular dysplasia. Inferior wall of right ventricle showing almost total replacement of myocardium by adipose tissue.

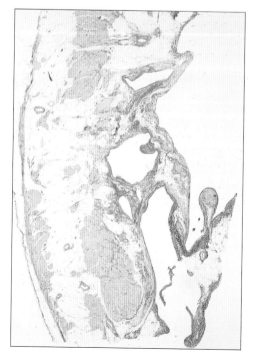

Fig. 12.20 Histological aspect of ventricular wall in arrhythmogenic right ventricular dysplasia. Islands of myocardium are still present amidst fat tissue. (EVG stain.)

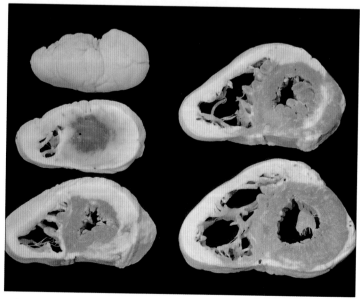

Fig. 12.21 Arrhythmogenic right ventricular dysplasia. Cross sections of heart show extension of fat tissue into left ventricular myocardium, apart from extensive right ventricular involvement.

13 ACQUIRED CONDITIONS PRIMARILY AFFECTING PRESSURE/VOLUME LOAD

Among the cardiac conditions that primarily affect the pressure or volume load of the heart, valvar pathology ranks highest. In general terms of functional pathology, a valve can either be stenotic or insufficient, although a combination of the two is common. Valvar pathology on the left side of the heart may have a profound effect on the pulmonary vascular bed as well as affecting the right side of the heart (see Section 3). Abnormalities of the valves of the right heart may also affect the left heart, but usually to a lesser extent.

The types of prevailing valvar abnormalities differ from one part of the world to another and even within the West important shifts in prevalence have occurred over the past decades. Rheumatic valvar disease, for instance, has become less of a problem, whereas conditions such as prolapse of the mitral valve and age-related valvar diseases (see also Chapter 15) have gained in significance. Infective endocarditis, in previous decades a disease of young people with pre-existing cardiac pathology, has veered markedly towards the elderly patient without a history of heart disease. Iatrogenic cardiac disease, moreover, can no longer be considered a bagatelle.

IMMUNE-RELATED VALVAR HEART DISEASE

Under this heading we will discuss auto-allergic diseases such as systemic lupus erythematosus, rheumatoid arthritis and rheumatic fever. The pathology that results from the latter is collectively known as rheumatic valvar disease.

Rheumatic valvar disease

In the Western part of the world the significance of rheumatic disease is declining thanks to early prevention, although in many other parts of the world rheumatic fever remains prevalent and is still a major disabling condition. Among the auto-allergic diseases rheumatic fever is the most important as far as the heart is concerned. It is generally considered that, following an infection of the throat, auto-allergy is elicited by cross-reactivity between the membrane antigen determinants of ß-haemolytic streptococci, and certain proteins present in the heart. Recurrent attacks may thus produce repeated episodes of injury and repair. When located in the valves, these eventually result in scar formation and functional impairment. Interstitial myocardial fibrosis is of less clinical significance than the valvar malformations that eventually ensue.

In the acute stage, the injury causes an inflammatory reaction dominated by oedema. Fibrinoid necrosis of connective tissues and a cellular reaction may occur. The valvitis leads to verrucous deposits of fibrin along the line of closure of the leaflets (Fig. 13.1), indicating a process of traumatic injury secondary to forceful closure. This observation is relevant since the deformities that eventually lead to cardiac disability show preference for those valves that sustain the highest pressures. The frequency with which the different valves are said to be involved depends upon the type of investigation. Pathological studies usually report a higher incidence than do clinical reports. Nevertheless, the mitral valve is by far the most commonly affected, although the combined involvement of mitral and aortic valves is the most frequent.

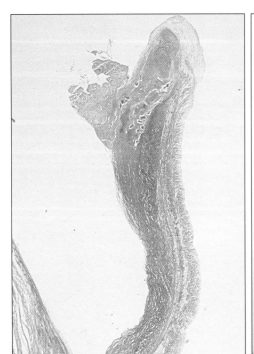
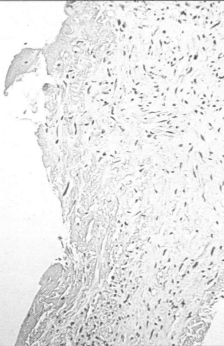

Fig. 13.1 Histology of the aortic valve in acute rheumatic fever: (left) verrucous fibrin depositions at site of closure; (right) fibrinoid necrosis with cellular reaction. E-VG (left), H&E (right) stains. By courtesy of Dr C.C. Lenox.

The healed stage of rheumatic valvar disease (often referred to as 'chronic') is characterized by deformities representing a longstanding and continuous process of injury and repair.

The mitral valvar apparatus is usually seriously affected by fibrosis of the leaflets, fusion of commissures and fibrosis of cords with obliteration of the intercordal spaces (Fig. 13.2). As a consequence, the normally high mobile valve is transformed into a rigid, irregularly thickened and funnel-like structure. The principal orifice is narrowed and displaced into the left ventricular cavity. These features are well demonstrated in a long-axis section (Fig. 13.3).

The degree and extent of the changes varies from one individual to another. Cases can occur with retraction of the leaflets as the dominant pathology (Fig. 13.4) and insufficiency as the main clinical feature, whilst in other cases, commissural and cordal fusion dominate the pathology (Fig. 13.5), with stenosis the prevailing clinical consequence. In advanced cases with extreme commissural fusion and funnel-like adherence of leaflets and cords, particularly when further aggravated by valvar calcifications, simple commissurotomy brings little relief. The same applies to the long term effects of balloon valvoplasty, which basically can be considered to represent commissurotomy.

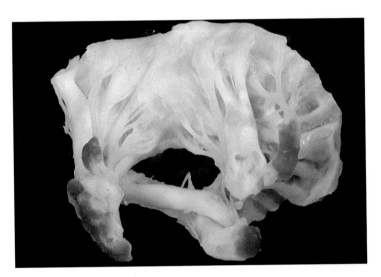

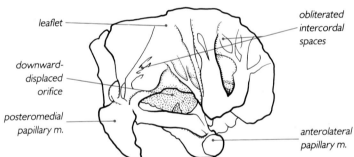

Fig. 13.2 Resected and stenotic valve in chronic rheumatic valve disease showing fibrosis of leaflets and cords and fusion of commissures.

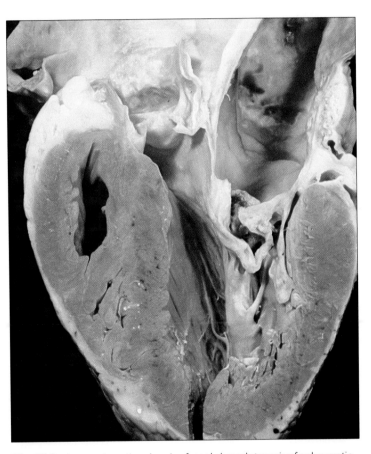

Fig. 13.3 Long-axis section showing funnel-shaped stenosis of a rheumatic mitral valve.

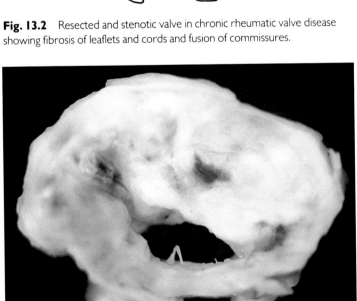

Fig. 13.4 Atrial view of resected rheumatic mitral valve showing retraction of the mural leaflet as the dominating feature producing insufficiency.

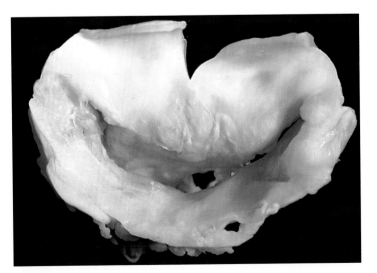

Fig. 13.5 Atrial view of resected rheumatic mitral valve showing commissural and cordal fusion as the dominating pathology producing stenosis.

In many instances, the basal part of the leaflet adjoining the aortic root is less affected and still pliable and transparent (Fig. 13.6). This part of the leaflet may thus produce a convexity towards the left atrium and, for a long time, ensure efficient closure of the valve despite advanced rheumatic involvement

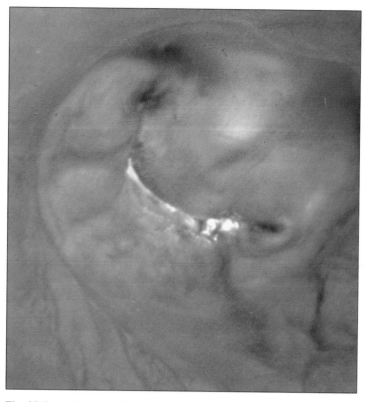

Fig. 13.6 Atrial view of rheumatic mitral valve showing its crescent-shaped orifice. Transillumination from the ventricular side shows the preserved transparency of the basal aspect of the aortic leaflet.

with retraction of the leaflets. The corvexity should not be confused with prolapse (see below). Even in the presence of severe disease the shape of the aortic leaflet is essentially preserved, whereas the usual scalloping of the mural leaflet tends to disappear, leaving a semicircular fibrous shelf (Fig. 13.6). The growth of relatively large-calibre vessels into the leaflet illustrates the inflammatory nature of the valvar deformity (Fig. 13.7). Contrary to common belief, however, this feature is not diagnostic of rheumatic disease.

Clinical rheumatic disease of the mitral valve, itself produced over a long period of time, is usually associated with an enlarged left atrium. In cases of longstanding insufficiency the left atrium can be huge. The endocardium is often corrugated and calcifications are common (Fig. 13.8). The deformed valve may show dystrophic calcifications with a preference for the commissural sites, in particular the posteromedial commissure. The calcific deposits may invade the junctional attachment of the leaflets and the adjacent myocardium, and a calcified rheumatic valve may coexist with so-called calcified mitral ring (see Chapter 15). The calcific deposits occur predominantly on the ventricular side of the valve, but occasionally they erode the atrial surface (Fig. 13.9). Thrombosis adherent to such exposed calcifications is common and may be a source of thromboembolism. Restenosis following commissurotomy carries a high incidence of dystrophic calcification as a late complication. Calcific embolization can also occur, although rarely with mitral valve disease. The dilated left atrium can be largely filled with mural thrombosis but the pulmonary venous channels are usually preserved (Fig. 13.10). Massive left atrial thrombosis occurs more frequently with mitral stenosis than with mitral insufficiency. Thrombus of the left atrial appendage is almost always present when rheumatic mitral disease is complicated by atrial fibrillation. Thromboembolism may then become a serious complication.

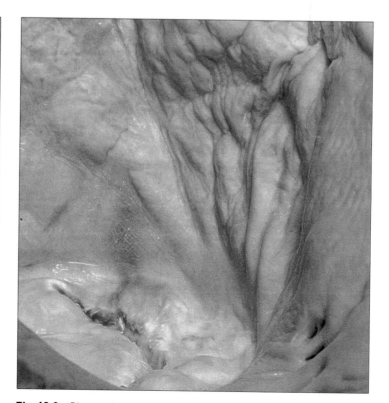

Fig. 13.7 Rheumatic mitral valve with extensive vascularity. The vessels have been injected with barium.

Fig. 13.8 Rheumatic stenosis of the mitral valve and huge dilatation of the left atrium with corrugated endocardium containing calcifications.

Right ventricular hypertrophy is a common cardiac consequence, being particularly outspoken in hearts with pure mitral stenosis. In such cases the marked right ventricular hypertrophy contrasts strikingly with the non-hypertrophied left ventricle (Fig. 13.11) and is followed by right atrial dilatation. Atrial fibrillation is a common, though non-specific, clinical finding.

The aortic valve exhibits similar changes to those in the mitral valve. The pathology is dominated by fibrosis and commissural fusion, often eccentric in nature (Fig. 13.12) and calcification may accompany these changes. Eccentric commissural fusion may mimic a congenitally bicuspid aortic valve with a raphé in the conjoined leaflet. However, close inspection will usually

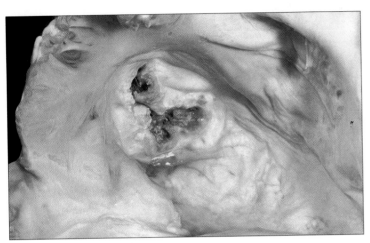

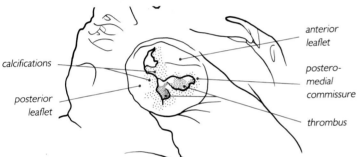

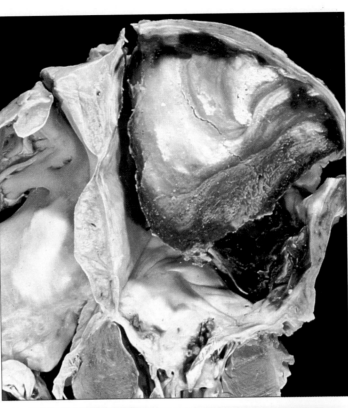

Fig. 13.9   Rheumatic mitral valve showing gross calcifications extending onto adjacent leaflets. There is adherent thrombosis.

Fig. 13.10   Four-chamber section showing dilated left atrium largely filled with mural thrombosis. The pulmonary venous channels were preserved.

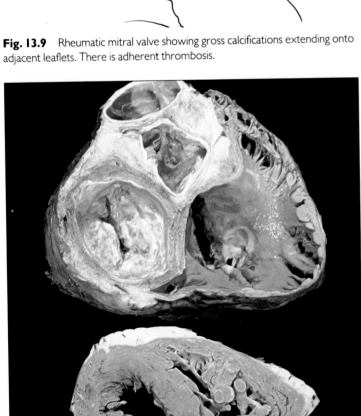

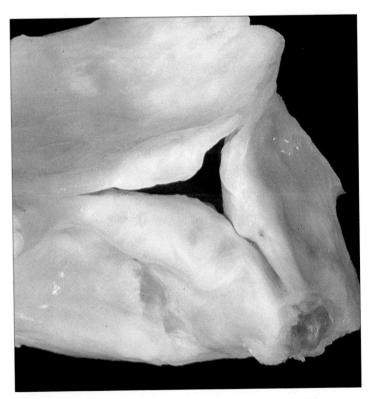

Fig. 13.11   Isolated rheumatic stenosis of the mitral valve and marked hypertrophy of the right ventricle contrasts with non-hypertrophied left ventricular wall.

Fig. 13.12   Aortic aspect of resected aortic valve with fibrosis of the leaflets and eccentric commissural fusion with calcifications – signs of rheumatic disease.

reveal the two leaflets to be 'glued' together (Fig. 13.13). Histological sections of the commissural site show extensive fibrosis as the 'glue' (Fig. 13.14). The nature of these changes is as in the apparatus of the mitral valve, with friction between different components playing an important role.

In longstanding cases the aortic valve becomes more heavily calcified (Fig. 13.15), often with a corrugated surface and adherent thrombosis. The gross aspect of this end-stage pathology is non-specific. So-called isolated calcific aortic stenosis occurring on the basis of degenerative diseases may have a similar appearance.

The tricuspid valve, when affected, shows fibrosis of the leaflets and fusion of commissures (Fig. 13.16) very similar to rheumatic lesions affecting the mitral valve. Cordal fusion, however, is not a striking feature and calcification is exceptional. In the Western world, tricuspid stenosis is exceptionally rare as the dominating clinical feature. Tricuspid insufficiency, on the other hand, is much more common. The combination of leaflet retraction in the setting of a hypertrophied and dilated right ventricle consequent to left-sided valvar pathology may underlie this particular complication.

The pulmonary valve is only rarely involved. In the event that it is, the changes are similar to those seen in the aortic valve. The incidence of pulmonary valvar disease is probably greatly influenced by the pressure of sustained pulmonary hypertension consequent to left heart disease.

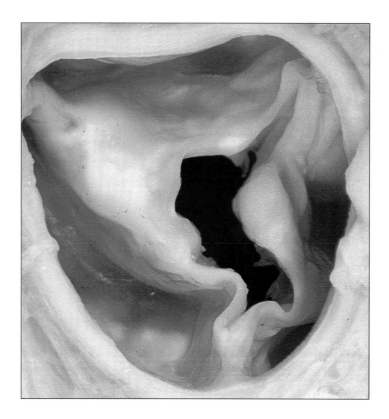

Fig. 13.13 Aortic aspect of rheumatic aortic valve showing eccentric commissural fusion. The two leaflets can still be identified.

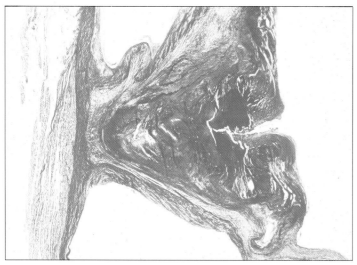

Fig. 13.14 Histological section through affected commissure showing dense fibrous tissue interposed between two leaflets at the site of commissural fusion. E-VG stain.

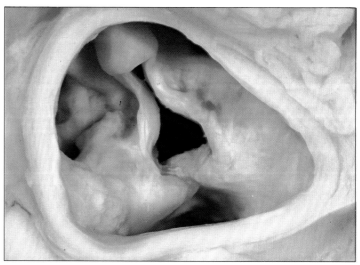

Fig. 13.15 Rheumatic aortic valve with involvement of all three commissures and more extensive calcifications affecting commissural sites as well as extending onto the leaflets.

Rheumatoid arthritis

This disease also belongs to the category of auto-allergic diseases and is characterized by the occurrence of antibodies against altered IgG. The aetiology is unknown. Like other generalized auto-allergic diseases, different organs may be involved, usually via an immune complex vasculitis, although whether this mechanism is involved in the pathogenesis of rheumatoid valvar disease remains unclear. Rheumatoid valvar disease most commonly affects the mitral valve. Involvement of the aortic valve is the next most common, followed by combined involvement of the aortic and mitral valves. Lesions of the tricuspid valve, or involvement of all four valves, are exceedingly rare. The valvar lesions are largely confined to the fibrous layers and consist either of small granulomatous lesions or areas of fibrinoid necrosis with a granulomatous marginal zone (Fig. 13.17). Fibrosis could ensue in these patients, particularly following sustained treatment with steroids.

Ankylosing spondylitis, considered a variant of rheumatoid arthritis, leads to dilatation of the aortic root and, hence, to aortic regurgitation. The valvar lesions are usually secondary to the altered haemodynamics.

Systemic lupus erythematosus

Systemic lupus erythematosus is a generalized auto-allergic disease, characterized by the occurrence of antibodies directed against a variety of auto-antigens, such as DNA, RNA, lymphocytes, complement factors and intracellular organelles. The aetiology is unknown. Pathology is induced mainly by depositions of immune complexes, and many organ systems may be involved, including the heart. One of the most important cardiac effects is acute pericarditis (see Chapter 14), but myocardial lesions also occur (see Section 5).

The pathology is dominated by a distinctive type of valvar and mural endocarditis, so-called Libman–Sacks endocarditis. This is characterized by the presence of verrucous greyish lesions along the closure line of the valves, as well as being draped along the undersurface and extending onto the mural endocardium. The lesions are composed of aggregates of fibrin and platelets. The mitral valve is most frequently affected, with the tricuspid valve a close second. Despite the fact that valvar involvement is common, haemodynamically significant lesions are rare. When reported, however, aortic and mitral insufficiency is the dominant feature. Mitral stenosis can occur, while haemodynamically

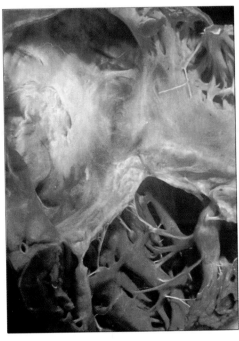
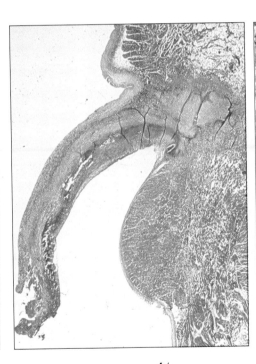
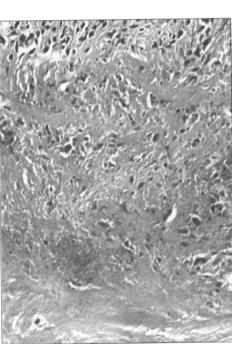

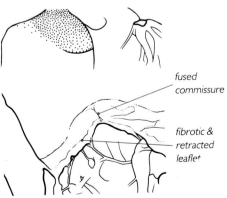

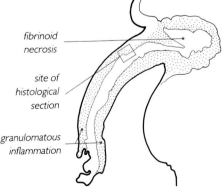

Fig. 13.16 Rheumatic involvement of the tricuspid valve includes fibrosis and retraction of leaflets together with commissural fusion. The cordal abnormalities are less striking.

fused commissure

fibrotic & retracted leaflet

fibrinoid necrosis

site of histological section

granulomatous inflammation

Fig. 13.17 Histology of mitral valve in rheumatoid arthritis (left), fibrinoid necrosis of the fibrous layer with granulomatous marginal zone seen in detail (right). H&E stain. By courtesy of Dr F. Eulderink.

significant aortic stenosis, due to extensive thrombotic vegetations, has been described. Bacterial endocarditis may complicate the valvar lesions and spontaneous valve perforation can occur (Fig. 13.18).

The histology is characterized by fibrinoid degeneration of collagen with a marginal cellular reaction composed mainly of mononuclear inflammatory cells and fibroblasts. In itself, this is a non-specific reaction, and beyond the active stage the lesions may heal leaving fibrous scars. Treatment with steroids may change the pathologic spectrum of the cardiac lesions. Healed lesions characterized by fibrosis would dominate the picture instead of the classically described exuberant multivalvar vegetations.

FLOPPY MITRAL VALVE

In the West the waning clinical relevance of rheumatic valve disease as a cause of mitral insufficiency has led to waxing interest in an anomaly best designated as 'floppy mitral valve'. The lesion is known by a variety of names such as myxomatous mitral valve, ballooning or billowing mitral valve, prolapse of the mitral valve, mitral valve click syndrome and Barlow's syndrome.

Inaccurate definitions have led to much confusion, particularly since prolapse of the mitral valve leaflets can occur in a variety of conditions, such as ischaemic heart disease and hypertrophic cardiomyopathy. The terms 'idiopathic' and 'primary versus

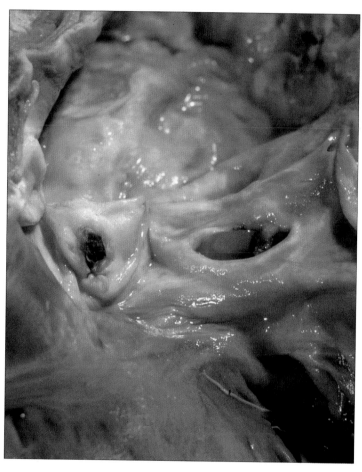

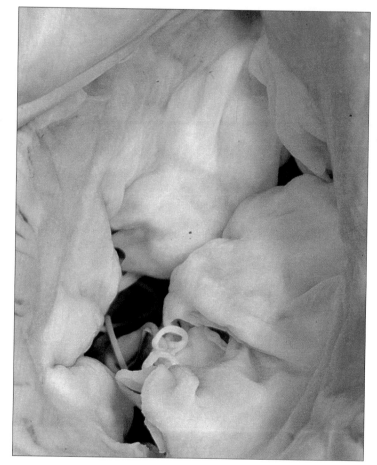

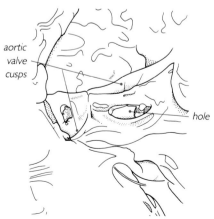

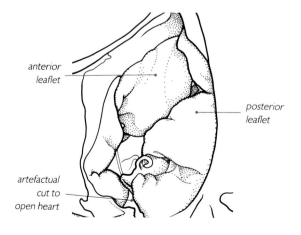

Fig. 13.18 Gross aspect of the aortic valve in a patient who had suffered systemic lupus erythematosus. The cusps show 'punched out' holes; infectious endocarditis was ruled out.

Fig. 13.19 Left atrial view of floppy mitral valve.

secondary' have been introduced to distinguish between these various forms of prolapse.

In the present context, the term 'floppy mitral valve' is used for an abnormality in the absence of a clearly identifiable aetiology. In general terms, the mitral valve shows redundant leaflets with domes projecting towards the left atrial cavity (Fig. 13.19). The domes may show a distinct overshoot producing an anatomical substrate for mitral insufficiency (Fig. 13.20). Not all mitral valves designated as floppy by the pathologist will necessarily have been insufficient during life (Fig. 13.21). Almost any part of the leaflets may be affected, although the lesion tends to concentrate around the posteromedial commissure, leaving the

anterolateral commissure and its bordering leaflets less affected (Fig. 13.21). The deformities are usually most pronounced in the mural leaflet (Fig. 13.22). The dome-shaped deformities should not be confused with the 'hoods' that occur naturally as atrial convexities of the leaflets between the sites of cordal anchorage.

The cords supporting the floppy leaflets are often attenuated, although in some areas the cords may be thickened. An abnormal lacework of cords is often present at the site of anchorage, leaving large areas of leaflet devoid of proper cordal insertions (Fig. 13.23), with cordal rupture the most common complication

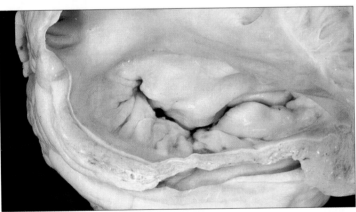

Fig. 13.20 Floppy mitral valve with overshoot of the middle scallop of the posterior leaflet unequivocally producing insufficiency.

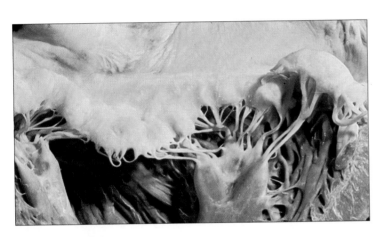

Fig. 13.21 Floppy leaflets located around the posteromedial commissure of the mitral valve but without overshoot.

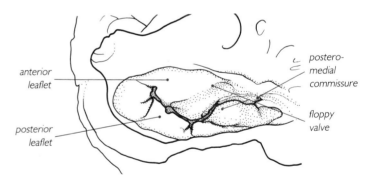

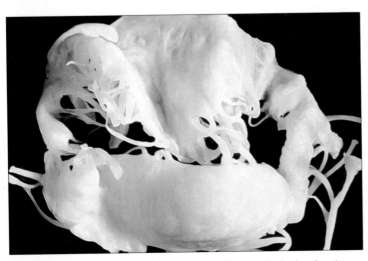

Fig. 13.22 Atrial aspect of surgically resected floppy mitral valve showing gross prolapse of middle scallop.

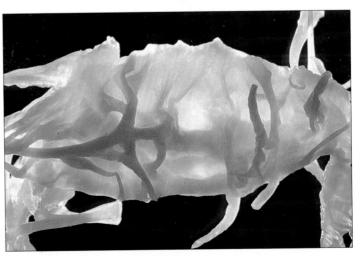

Fig. 13.23 Ventricular view of a surgically excised floppy mural leaflet of the mitral valve showing abnormally textured cords.

(Fig. 13.24). The typical history in such cases is that of a patient known for some time to have signs of a floppy mitral valve in whom a sudden onset of aggravation of mitral insufficiency occurs in the absence of signs of infectious disease. Depending upon the overall nature of the deficient cordal support, rupture may lead to minor (Fig. 13.25) or major (Fig. 13.26) prolapse.

Floppy mitral valve has been described as the underlying disease in patients with transient ischaemic cerebral attacks, although the mechanism involved remains unclear. It has also been associated with angina pectoris in the presence of normal coronary arteries with ventricular arrhythmias and sudden death.

Another association that cannot be accounted for by chance is the combination of floppy mitral valve and large atrial septal defects within the oval fossa. The abnormality of the valve tends to be confined to the area of the posteromedial commissure, suggesting lack of support as the underlying mechanism. Floppy mitral valve is also a common finding in patients with Marfan's syndrome (Fig. 13.27).

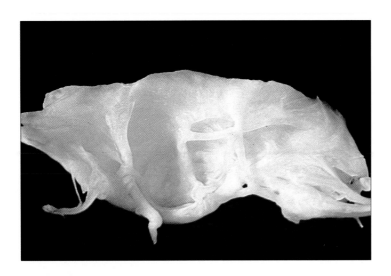

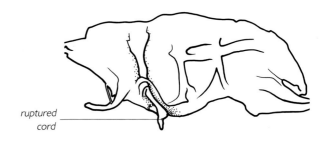

Fig. 13.24 Ventricular view of a surgically excised mural leaflet from a floppy mitral valve showing cordal rupture.

ruptured
cord

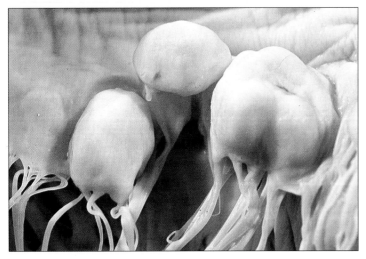

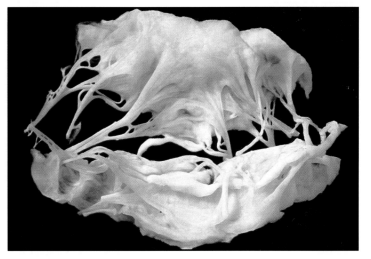

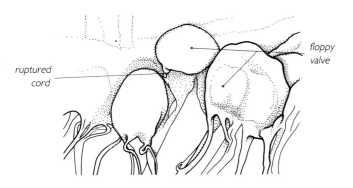

ruptured
cord

floppy
valve

prolapse of
mural
leaflet

ruptured
cordae

Fig. 13.25 Cordal rupture in a floppy mitral valve showing minor prolapse.

Fig. 13.26 Left ventricular aspect of surgically excised specimen of floppy mitral valve with cordal rupture and major prolapse of the mural leaflet.

The aetiology and pathogenesis of floppy mitral valve remain controversial. Valves thus affected show an excessive accumulation of glycosaminoglycans (Fig. 13.28). The atrial aspect, moreover, may show a thickening composed of layers of collagen fibres (Fig. 13.29) secondary to regurgitant flow and abnormal friction. Different opinions emerge regarding the interpretation of these findings. Most investigators take the myxomatous change as the primary underlying cause of idiopathic mitral valve prolapse. In this respect, Marfan's syndrome serves as the paradigm.

The myxoid change observed histologically, however, could also represent an expression of a secondary event, such as prolonged or undue stress on the valvar apparatus causing accelerated collagen degradation. The observation of a wide spectrum of cordal arrangements in normal hearts, rendering parts of the leaflets less well supported than others, together with the observation that resected specimens of floppy mitral valve exhibit abnormalities in cordal anchorage, endorse the concept of a secondary mechanism as at least one of the possibilities (Fig. 13.30).

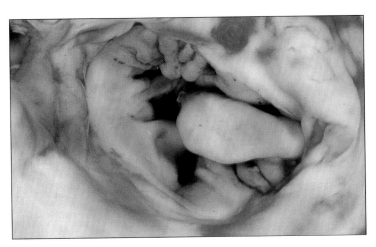

Fig. 13.27 Floppy mitral valve in infant with Marfan's syndrome.

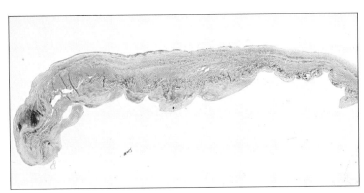

Fig. 13.28 Histological section of floppy leaflet showing excessive accumulation of glycosaminoglycans.

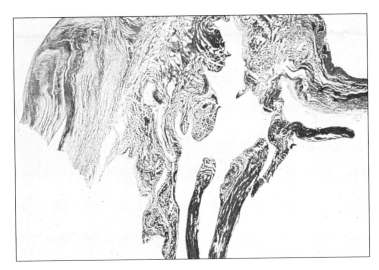

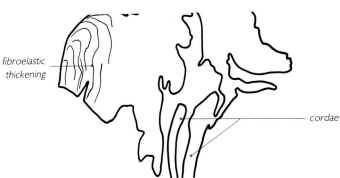

Fig. 13.29 Histological section of prolapsed leaflet of the mitral valve showing excessive fibroelastic tissue at atrial aspect. E-VG stain.

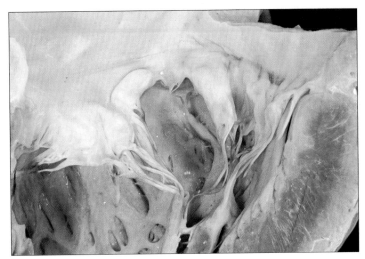

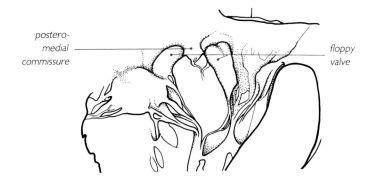

Fig. 13.30 Floppy mitral valve in which the affected segment, centring around the posteromedial commissure, has almost no cordal support.

INFECTIVE ENDOCARDITIS

The term 'infective' is preferred over 'bacterial' endocarditis since it is well acknowledged that a wide variety of organisms may cause this disease. An important shift has taken place in recent years regarding the type of patient involved. In the 'old' days, infective endocarditis particularly affected patients with rheumatic valvar or congenital heart disease. Presently, the average age of the patient has markedly risen and, usually, there is no past history of heart disease. Instead, degenerative valvar changes play an important role in elderly patients, not only in cases with overt changes such as calcific aortic valvar disease or calcified mitral ring (see below), but also in patients with apparently no valvar abnormalities. The process of 'wear and tear' that affects the tissues of valves over the years may render them susceptible to infection, particularly when organisms invade the elderly patient with an altered immune-defense capacity. In valves showing such 'wear and tear' changes, the endothelial surface of the valves is altered and the line of closure

often accentuated (Fig. 13.31). More detailed histological studies often reveal adherent aggregates of fibrin and platelets. Such lesions may thus form a nidus for circulating microorganisms and form the foundation for infective endocarditis in an apparently normal valve (see also Chapter 15). At present, it is also important to consider iatrogenic causes for infective endo-carditis. The number of patients with intracardiac pacemaker electrodes and prosthetic valves (see below) is ever increasing. Furthermore, since the longevity of patients with congenital heart disease has improved considerably, thanks to corrective and palliative cardiac surgery, the risk of acquiring infective endocarditis is a constant threat in this set of patients. The problem of the increasing number of drug addicts in whom infective endocarditis is a common and often fatal complication must also be faced. Whatever the background, the source of infection is not always clear. Dental and gingival infections, infections of the respiratory and urinary tracts, as well as skin infections, are still the most important primary sites. The list of micro-organisms able to produce endocarditis is enormous. For

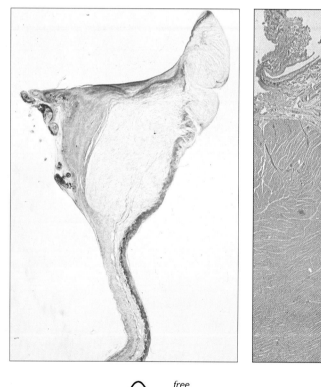

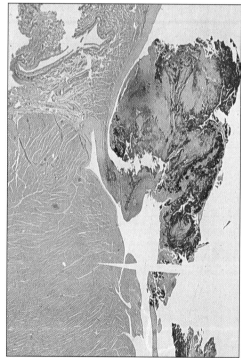

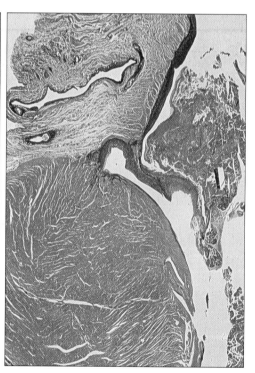

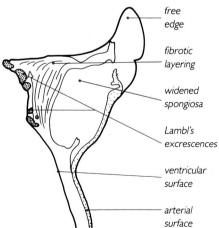

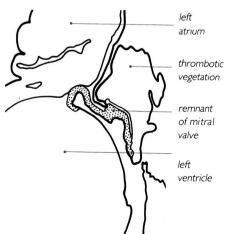

Fig. 13.31 Histological section of a leaflet from the aortic valve showing surface alterations at the site of closure. E-VG stain.

Fig. 13.32 Histological section showing virtual destruction of a leaflet of the mitral valve by staphylococci. (Left) Gram stain; (right) E-VG stain.

practical purposes every micro-organism (including viruses), thus far reported has the potential to produce endocarditis.

Infective endocarditis predominantly affects the valves. Mural endocarditis usually occurs as an extension from a diseased valve. Pre-existent mural endocardial changes, such as those evoked by jet or cordal friction, may occasionally underlie a primary endocarditic lesion. The left side of the heart is most commonly affected, the mitral valve having a slightly higher incidence of primary infection than the aortic valve. Tricuspid involvement is infrequent and infection of the pulmonary valve is extremely rare.

Basically, infective endocarditis is a disease that destroys the valve (Fig. 13.32). The type of micro-organisms involved, the immune state of the host, and the speed with which the disease is properly diagnosed and treated all determine the clinical course and outcome. For these reasons, a division into acute and subacute endocarditis is nowadays of less significance. If left untreated, the prognosis is largely determined by the damage present when the disease is controlled. The complications of infective endocarditis can thus be classified into destructive effects on the valve, invasive effects onto neighbouring cardiac structures and septic embolic effects. A late consequence of infective endocarditis occurs when the immune complexes evoked produce generalized vasculitis, with renal involvement then being a particular threat.

Infective endocarditis of the mitral valve tends to occur at its atrial surface, initially at the site of coaptation of the leaflets (Fig. 13.33). This is also the natural site for age-related changes. A thrombotic mass usually adheres to the site of infection and often contains vast colonies of micro-organisms (Fig. 13.32). This is one of the reasons why high doses of intravenous antibiotics are mandatory if they are to be effective at those sites. The infection may easily spread onto adjacent parts of the leaflet (Fig. 13.34) as well as onto the cords. Cordal destruction can then lead to prolapse of the affected leaflet and massive mitral insufficiency (Fig. 13.34). Eventually, the central part of the leaflet may be completely destroyed, leaving a hole amidst infected tissue (Fig. 13.35). When cured at this stage, subsequent valve replacement is almost always necessary (Fig. 13.36).

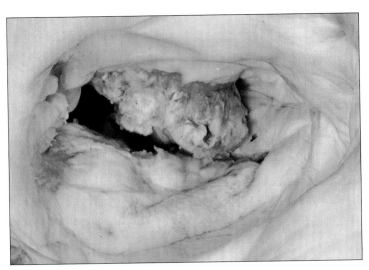

Fig. 13.33 Infective endocarditis of the mitral valve showing destruction of atrial aspect, predominantly on the aortic leaflet, with adherent thrombosis.

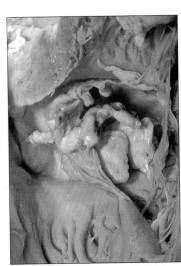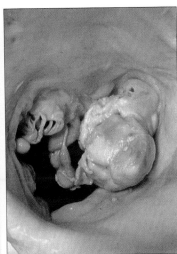

Fig. 13.34 Infective endocarditis of the mitral valve with cordal rupture: (left) left ventricular view; (right) left atrial aspect with prolapsing leaflets at the posteromedial commissure.

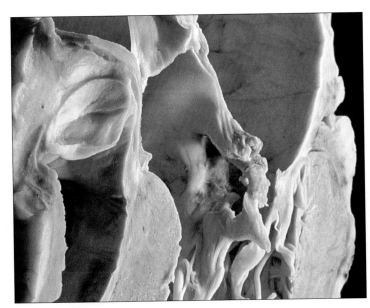

Fig. 13.35 Infective endocarditis: destruction of a leaflet of the mitral valve in active stage with defect amidst infected tissue.

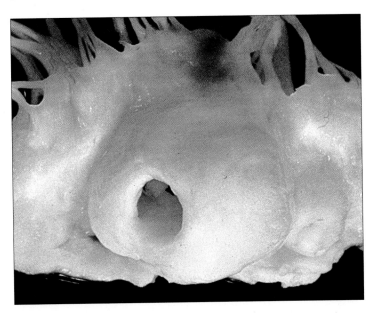

Fig. 13.36 Infective endocarditis of the mitral valve: surgically resected aortic leaflet with 'healed' lesion.

Calcific mitral ring is notably prone to infection (see also Chapter 15). The abnormal morphology and function renders the valve vulnerable to infection, for instance along its free edge and atrial surface (Fig. 13.37). The undersurface of the valve, which contains the degenerative calcific process (see Chapter 15), is also in jeopardy (Fig. 13.38). An infection at the annulus carries a poor prognosis since it may easily lead to the formation of an abscess (Fig. 13.39) which is often difficult to diagnose and treat. Pericarditis and death readily ensue. The development of pericarditis in any patient with clinical signs of an infectious disease of unknown nature should always raise the possibility of infective endocarditis.

Infective endocarditis of the aortic valve tends to occur on the ventricular aspect, again with the line of closure as the usual site (Figs 13.31, 13.40). For full understanding of the ensuing complications, it is necessary to have a complete knowledge of the topography of the aortic root (see also Chapter 1). The infection may spread anteriorly into the epicardium in the angle

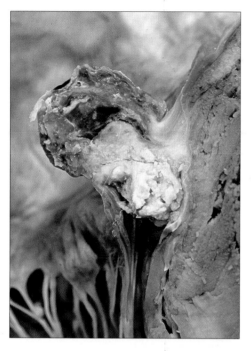

Fig. 13.37 Infective endocarditis on atrial aspect of the mural leaflet of the mitral valve complicating calcification of the ring.

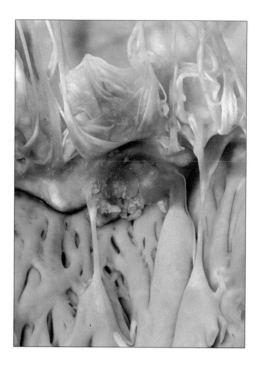

Fig. 13.38 Infective endocarditis at the site of calcification of the ring of the mitral valve showing the infected angle between the leaflet and the ventricular wall.

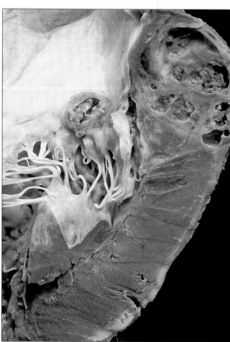

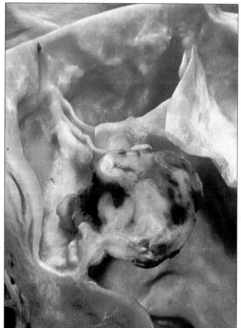

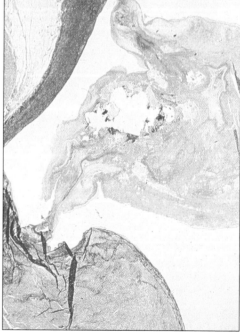

Fig. 13.39 Infective endocarditis: ring abscess of the mitral valve extending into epicardial fat tissue. The atrial aspect of the valve is eroded.

Fig. 13.40 Infective endocarditis of the aortic valve: (left) leaflet with thrombotic vegetation; (right) histology revealing destruction of the leaflet. E-VG stain.

between the right ventricular outflow tract and the zone of aortic–mitral valvar fibrous continuity (Fig. 13.41). It may give rise to an epicardial abscess in this location, with consequences as described for an abscess of the mitral ring. The infection may also spread into the right ventricular outflow tract (Fig. 13.42) as well as to the right (Fig. 13.43), and left atrial walls. The axis of atrioventricular conduction tissue may become involved, with production of heart block. The infection may then spread directly onto the ventricular surface of the adjoining mitral valvar leaflets (Fig. 13.44). Infective endocarditis of the aortic valve may thus result in infective mitral valvar disease. The occurrence of mitral insufficiency in the clinical setting of aortic valvar endocarditis is difficult to evaluate, even with sophisticated echocardiographic techniques, because aortic valvar endocarditis in itself can produce mitral insufficiency as a consequence of left ventricular dilatation and papillary muscle dysfunction.

The regurgitant and infected flow through a damaged aortic valve can lead to infection of the mitral valve at more remote sites (Fig. 13.45). Moreover, superficial spread on the left ventricular septal surface may lead to selective damage of the left

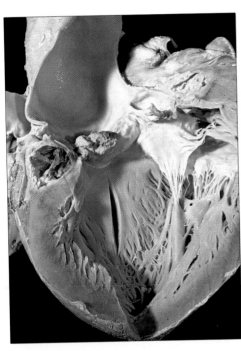

Fig. 13.41 Infective endocarditis of aortic valve leading to an abscess in the aortic root.

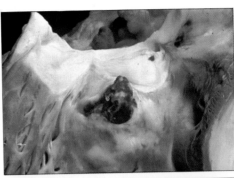

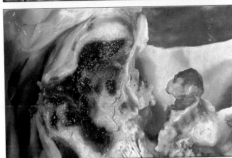

Fig. 13.42 Infective endocarditis of the aortic valve, which has perforated into the outflow tract of the right ventricle (upper); section showing root of spread (lower).

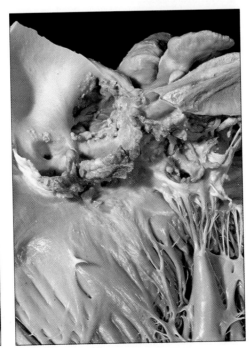

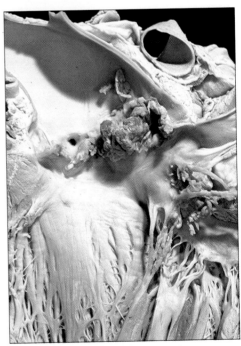

Fig. 13.43 Extension of infective endocarditis from the aortic valve into the right atrium.

Fig. 13.44 Direct spread of infective endocarditis from the aortic onto the mitral valve.

Fig. 13.45 Infective endocarditis: distant involvement of the aortic leaflet of the mitral valve and its cords. Note the unaffected segment of leaflet beneath the infected aortic valve.

bundle branches and, hence, to partial or complete left bundle branch block (Fig. 13.46). As with infective endocarditis of the mitral valve, the infection may have destroyed the valve so extensively prior to cure that replacement becomes necessary. In some patients, the disease may take a fulminant course resistant to medical treatment which necessitates surgical replacement of the valve in the acute stage (Fig. 13.47). As previously stated, septic emboli are a frequent complication. In our autopsy series all patients who died in the setting of aortic valve infection had septic myocarditis (see also Section 5). This is particularly relevant when instituting appropriate treatment during life.

Infective endocarditis of the tricuspid valve is increasingly seen as a complication of drug addicts (Fig. 13.48). It is a misconception to think that other valves are not, or only rarely, affected in such individuals. Infection of the septal leaflet, which is located close to the membranous septum, may easily spread to the atrioventricular node and penetrating atrioventricular bundle. Disturbances of atrioventricular conduction may thus appear as an early complication. The signs and symptoms of infection of the tricuspid valve are different from those that occur with left-sided endocarditis. Septic embolization into the lungs cause recurrent pulmonary infections and should alert to infection of the tricuspid valve, particularly in young individuals.

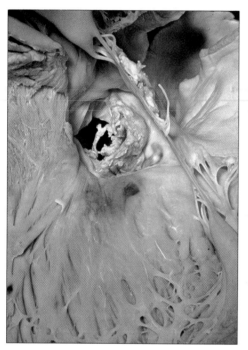

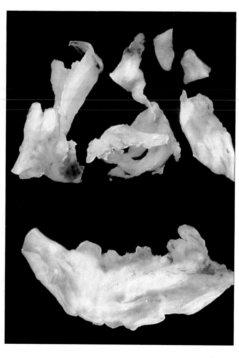

Fig. 13.47 Surgically removed aortic valve showing acute phase of bacterial endocarditis.

Fig. 13.46 Infective endocarditis of the aortic valve spreading onto the left ventricular surface and producing left bundle branch block. Note involvement of the mitral valve.

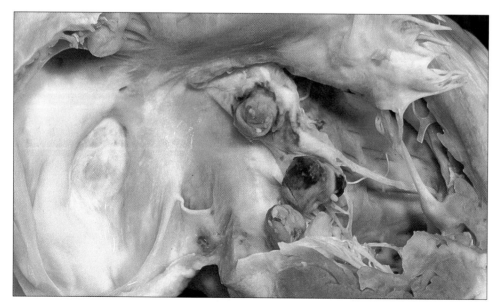

Fig. 13.48 Infective endocarditis of tricuspid valve in a known heroin addict.

DEGENERATIVE PATHOLOGY OF THE AORTIC VALVE

Degenerative disease of the aortic valve is of major clinical importance. The lesions found are almost always heavily calcified (Fig. 13.49), hence the often used term 'isolated calcific aortic valvar' disease. In approximately half of the patients, the aortic valve is congenitally malformed, either bicuspid or (rarely) unicuspid in nature, while the remainder show a normal aortic valve with three leaflets. The common denominator in each category is degeneration of tissues as part of a process of wear and tear (see below). Dystrophic calcification occurs as a secondary effect (Fig. 13.50).

The unicuspid aortic valve is usually intrinsically stenotic and is one of the common forms of aortic stenosis in the very young (see also Section 4). Nevertheless, isolated stenosis of this type may occur in adult patients, the average age at which symptoms occur being approximately 40 years. The oldest patient we have seen with stenosis of a unicuspid valve was 69 years old.

Congenitally bicuspid aortic valves are not usually intrinsically stenotic. The vast majority of such valves encountered in adults and first recognized at autopsy contain gross calcific deposits.

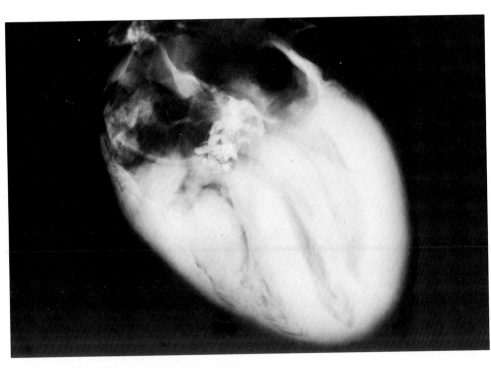

Fig. 13.49 Postmortem radiograph showing isolated pathology of the aortic valve.

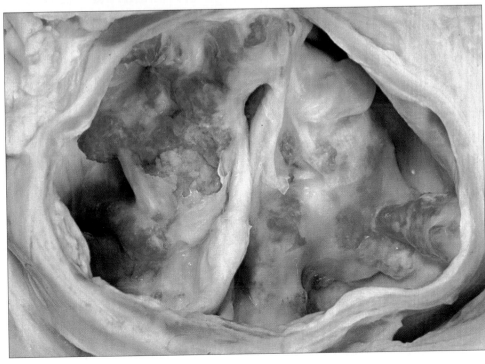

Fig. 13.50 Calcific stenosis due to a congenitally unicommissural and unicuspid valve in a male patient 69 years of age.

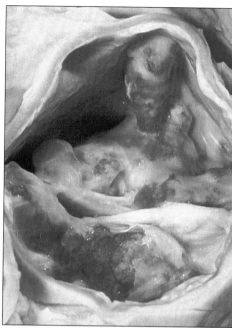

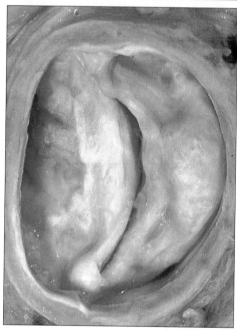

Fig. 13.51 Calcific stenosis in a bicuspid aortic valve with (upper) and without (lower) raphé.

These valves are rigid and non-pliable, irrespective of whether or not there is a conjoined leaflet with a raphé (Fig. 13.51).

As previously indicated, isolated pathology of the aortic valve also occurs in the aortic valve with three leaflets (Fig. 13.52), usually in patients over 65 years of age. The underlying degenerative changes in these valves again relate to a process of wear and tear. In the congenitally unicuspid and bicuspid aortic valves, enhanced degeneration is caused by the excess in pressure load on a single leaflet. In aortic valves with three leaflets, variations in size of the individual leaflets occur as a rule (Fig.

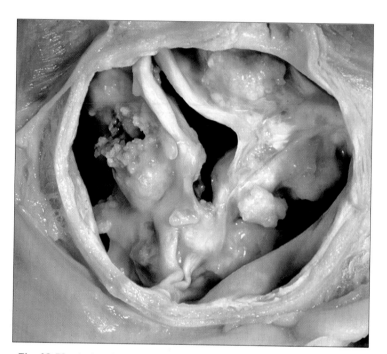

Fig. 13.52 Isolated calcific stenosis of the aortic valve in which the basically trifoliate nature is still recognizable; calcifications on the aortic sides of the leaflets are typical of age-related valvar pathology.

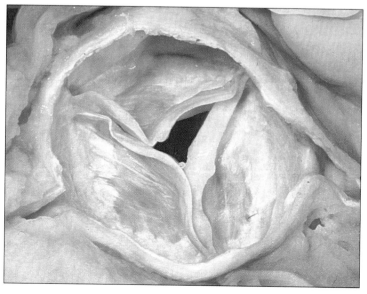

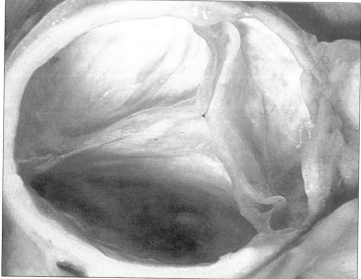

Fig. 13.53 Non-stenotic aortic valves: (left) three leaflets of almost equal sizes; (right) marked differences in sizes of the leaflets, the left coronary leaflet being tiny.

13.53). Hence, there is an unequal distribution of forces exerted on the leaflets both in diastole and systole. This fact provides the anatomical basis for enhanced 'wear and tear'.

Degenerative disease of the aortic valve usually results in stenosis and sudden death is well-known when the stenosis is severe. Death may be unexpected, particularly in the elderly patient, because the valvar pathology had passed unnoticed, once more emphasizing the enormous capacity of the myocardium for adaption (see also Chapter 3). Indeed, colossal left ventricular

hypertrophy is always present, but usually it is accompanied by signs of ischaemic myocardial damage (Fig. 13.54), thus providing a basis for sudden death.

Occasionally, signs of valvar insufficiency can be found in the presence of a heavily fibrotic and calcified valve (Fig. 13.55). Nonetheless, the incidence of valvar insufficiency as the dominant feature of degenerative disease of the aortic valve in elderly patients is low. Infective endocarditis, on the other hand, is by no means an infrequent complication (Fig. 13.56).

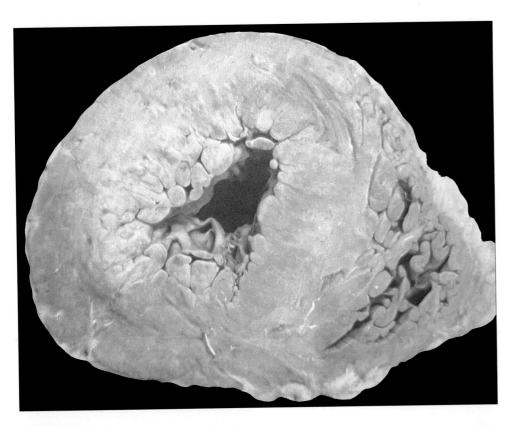

Fig. 13.54 Left ventricular hypertrophy in isolated calcific stenosis of the aortic valve exhibiting ischaemic changes confined mainly to the subendocardial zone.

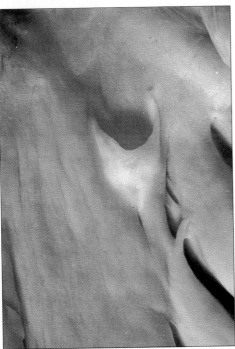

Fig. 13.55 Discrete endocardial fibrous pocket on the left ventricular aspect of the septum indicating insufficiency of the aortic valve.

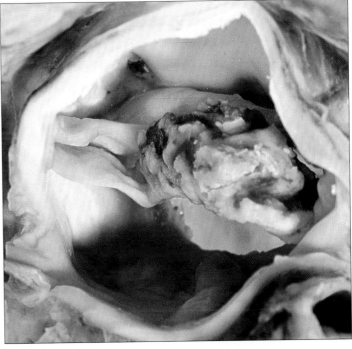

Fig. 13.56 Infective endocarditis of a congenitally bicuspid aortic valve with destruction of the base of the anterior leaflet. Calcifications are absent.

VALVAR AND ENDOCARDIAL PATHOLOGY: MISCELLANEOUS LESIONS

Acquired abnormalities of the cardiac valves and mural endo-cardium occur with a variety of diseases. It is beyond our scope to attempt a full account of all such abnormalities. Disease of the aortic valve producing significant symptoms may occur in patients suffering from such diverse diseases as syphilis, anky-losing spondylitis, Ehlers–Danlos syndrome or idiopathic and non-inflammatory dilatation of the aortic root. The common denominator in all these conditions is a widening of the aortic outflow tract at the level of attachment of the leaflets. Depending on the underlying disease, the leaflets themselves may either be transparent and non-pliable or somewhat fibrosed, but, in almost all instances, the free edges of the leaflets are rolled.

Syphilis

In the West, the chronic stage of syphilistic aortitis is of minor clinical significance at present. The disease is characterized by fibrosis and retraction of the leaflets with the commissures being slightly opened (Fig. 13.57, left). The aortic side of the commis-sure may be compromised by a prominent hyaline plaque (Fig. 13.57, right). Occasionally, these plaques fuse in circular fashion.

Non-inflammatory dilatation of the aortic root

The largest single cause of clinically significant aortic regurgita-tion is idiopathic and non-inflammatory dilatation of the aortic root. The disease is characterized by an increase in the diameter of the aortic root at the level of the peripheral attachments of the commissures (Fig. 13.58). The immediate cause of insuffi-ciency in these instances is prolapse of the leaflets which, in time, leads to fibrous thickening of their free edges (Fig. 13.59). Dilatation of the ascending aorta a few centimetres above this level is a common feature in the elderly and has no effect on the function of the aortic valve.

The pathogenesis of this important disease remains, as yet, enigmatic. The similarities with classical Marfan's disease has led to the supposition that non-inflammatory dilatation is a *formes fruste* of Marfan's syndrome. There is no firm scientific basis for this concept, despite the fact that isolated dilatation of the aortic

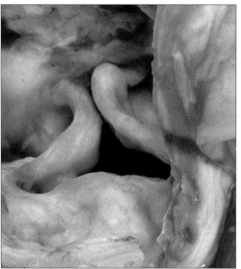

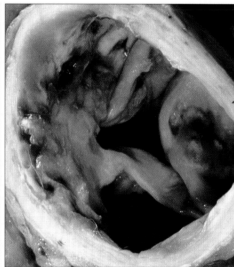

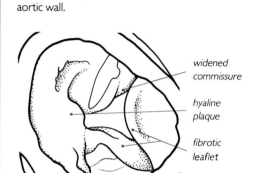

Fig. 13.57 Aortic root in syphilis: (left) typically widened commissures; (right) hyaline plaque on aortic wall.

widened commissure

hyaline plaque

fibrotic leaflet

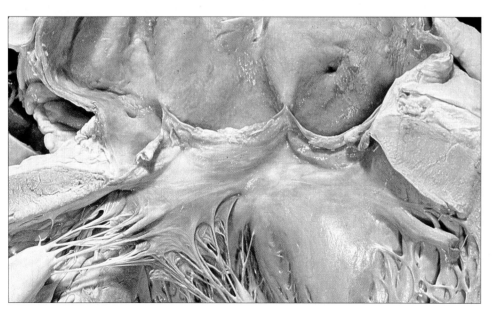

Fig. 13.58 Dilatation of the aortic root.

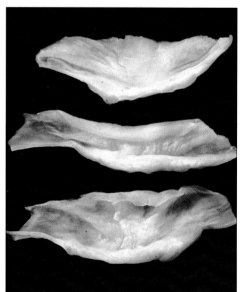

Fig. 13.59 Surgically excised leaflets of the aortic leaflets showing rolled free edges.

root may occur among relatives of patients with classical Marfan's disease. The histological findings in the aortic root show various degrees of fragmentation of elastic and collagen fibres, with accumulation of glycoaminoglycans. Such changes, from a histological point of view, indicate a process of injury and response of the aortic wall rather than being specific for any particular disease such as Marfan's syndrome. Since the disease shows a positive correlation with age, it is tempting to speculate that haemodynamic factors, associated with the altered geometry of the left ventricular outflow tract in the elderly, play a role in causing early degeneration of the supporting tissues.

Aortic valvar insufficiency may appear as a complicating feature in patients suffering from mitral insufficiency of various causes. Surgically excised valves from such cases show no appreciable pathology other than the changes mentioned above. A chronic and undue pull on the leaflets of the aortic valve via the aortic leaflet of the mitral valve in a dilated left ventricle may be the underlying pathogenetic mechanism.

Marfan's syndrome

Marfan's syndrome requires a full discussion because valvar pathology is one of its major manifestations. The disease is characterized by the production of an abnormally structured collagen-like protein and, hence, affects the integrity of the supportive tissues. These features play an important role in the pathogenesis of all its cardiovascular complications. Dissecting aneurysm of the aorta, dilatation of the aortic root and excessive laxity of the valvar leaflets leading to insufficiency are the most common abnormalities which affect the heart. Indeed, Marfan's syndrome is the classical example of prolapse of the leaflets of the mitral valve consequent to a floppy change (see Fig. 13.27). Usually, in addition to the floppy leaflets, the orifice of the mitral valve is markedly dilated. Aortic valvar insufficiency in these patients is then due to prolapse of the leaflets and dilatation of the aortic root, the leaflets showing extreme laxity (Fig. 13.60). Dissecting aneurysm of the ascending aorta may cause or aggravate aortic valvar insufficiency as a direct consequence (Fig. 13.61). Rupture of a dissecting aortic aneurysm into the pericardial cavity leads to cardiac tamponade. It is the second most frequent form of acute haemorrhagic pericardial effusion and death, following rupture of the free wall of the left ventricle (see Section 5). The dissecting haematoma may also cause narrowing of the orifices of the coronary arteries, particularly the right, with myocardial ischaemia and infarction as a result. This feature may compromise the clinical differentiation between dissecting aneurysm and acute myocardial infarction.

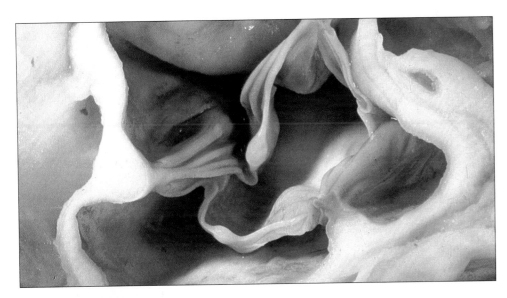

Fig. 13.60 Dilatation of the aortic root with floppy leaflets in Marfan's syndrome.

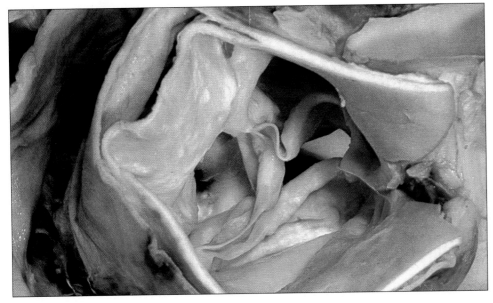

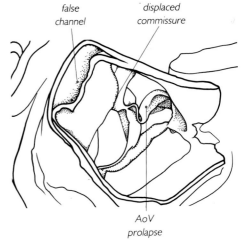

Fig. 13.61 Aortic dissection; an intramural haematoma has displaced the commissure leading to prolapse of leaflets and valvar insufficiency.

false channel

displaced commissure

AoV prolapse

Thrombotic endocarditis

Non-bacterial thrombotic endocarditis is another example of pathology afflicting the valves that may accompany a variety of diseases. The condition is known under various names of which 'non-bacterial thrombotic endocarditis' and 'marantic endocarditis' are the most widely used. The entity is characterized by verrucous and thrombotic vegetations adherent to the site of the closure of the valvar leaflets (Fig. 13.62). The mitral valve is most commonly affected, followed by the aortic valve and combined lesions involving the aortic and mitral valves. The tricuspid and pulmonary valves are rarely involved. The condition may easily be mistaken for infective endocarditis. Close observation, nonetheless, will show that the leaflets themselves are unaffected (Fig. 13.62) apart from alterations to their surface that occur with advanced age (see Chapter 15). Non-bacterial thrombotic endocarditis, however, may form the nidus for infection in the presence of circulating micro-organisms and when the immune status of the patient is compromised. The size and extent of the vegetations varies considerably. In some cases, the thrombotic mass may cover the full circumference of the line of closure, giving the impression of functional stenosis (Fig. 13.63).

Non-bacterial thrombotic endocarditis occurs predominantly in patients with a malignant disease. Tumours of the prostate, ovaries, pancreas, stomach and testis appear especially prone to producing these lesions, although they may coexist with any other tumour, as well as with non-tumorous diseases. As a rule, non-bacterial thrombotic endocarditis does not lead to clinical symptomatology. Its presence is usually an incidental autopsy finding. Thromboembolic complications, particularly in the cerebral vessels, can be the first sign of its presence. Similarly, thrombotic occlusions of the coronary arteries, both epicardial and intramural, may occur. Myocardial infarction is then a complication.

Non-bacterial thrombotic endocarditis is considered part of a more generalized 'pre-thrombotic state' of the blood, typified by a chronic form of intravascular clotting. The relation between hypercoagulability and malignancy is well founded. As a consequence, thrombotic arterial occlusions in these patients may be part of 'spontaneous' thrombosis rather than embolism, with the lesions on the valves as the prime source.

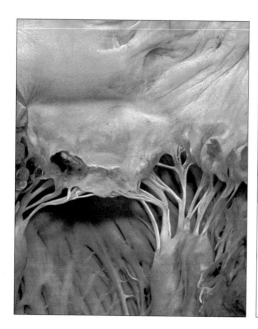
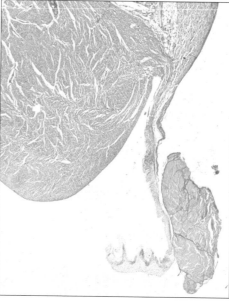

Fig. 13.62 Non-bacterial thrombotic endocarditis on the mitral valve: (left) thrombotic vegetations located along the line of closure; (right) histology shows thrombus adherent to an intact leaflet. E-VG stain.

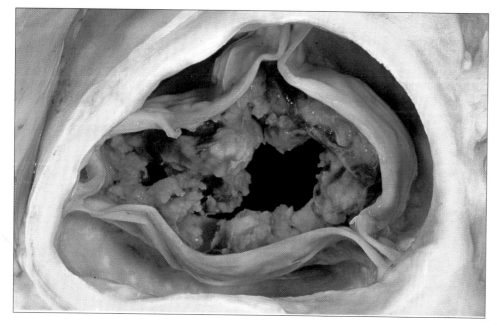

Fig. 13.63 Extensive non-bacterial thrombotic endocarditis narrowing the orifice of the aortic valve.

Carcinoid heart disease

The heart is involved in approximately half the patients who have a carcinoid tumour with metastatic spread. The right side of the heart is predominantly affected, although the mitral valve is involved occasionally. Carcinoid involvement of all four heart valves has been described in association with deficiency of the oval fossa. Carcinoid lesions appear as white plaques that cover the valves or the mural endocardium. The leaflets of the tricuspid (Fig. 13.64, left) and the pulmonary (Fig. 13.64, right) valves thus become markedly thickened, often with retraction and muscular ingrowth. The lesions are not usually confined to the leaflets but extend onto the tendinous cords and the mural endocardium related to the valves. Tricuspid insufficiency and pulmonary stenosis are common clinical findings.

Histologically, the carcinoid lesions are composed of relatively acellular 'young' fibrous tissue, sharply delineated from the underlying endocardium. The endocardium and valvar leaflets themselves are normal. The lesions are characteristically super-imposed on the ventricular aspect of the atrioventricular valves and the pulmonary side of the arterial valve (Fig. 13.65). The composition of the lesions may differ slightly from one case to another, varying from an acellular ground substance with a few spindle-shaped cells as the dominant feature to a predominantly collagenous aggregation, thus reflecting the age of the prolife-rative lesion. Ultrastructurally, the proliferating cells are shown to be smooth muscle-like cells or myofibroblasts. The patho-genesis of the carcinoid lesions remains unclear as yet.

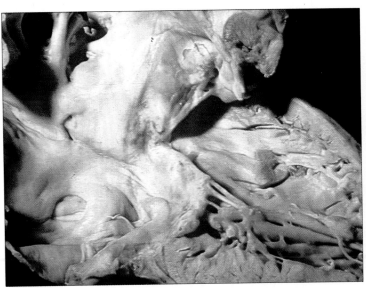

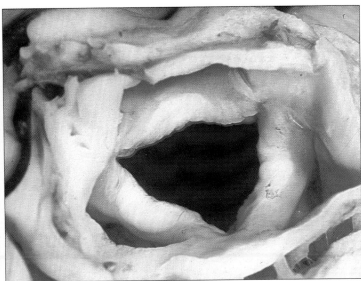

Fig. 13.64 Carcinoid heart disease: marked thickening of the leaflets of the tricuspid (left) and pulmonary valves (right).

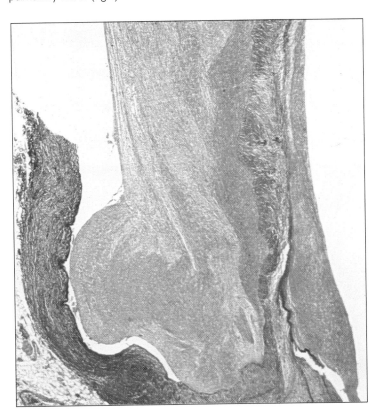

Fig. 13.65 Histological section of a leaflet from the pulmonary valve in carcinoid heart disease showing deposition of fibrous tissue, mainly localized in the sinus; the leaflet is basically normal. E-VG stain.

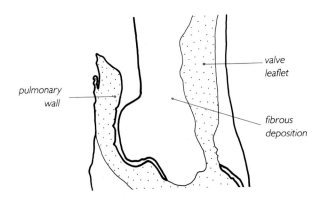

PATHOLOGY OF PROSTHETIC VALVES

The success of replacement of cardiac valves is greatly influenced by pre-existent pathology. Conditions such as a heavily calcified valve with extensive myocardial involvement, or massive myocardial hypertrophy with a small ventricle, may necessitate adjustments of technique during surgery. The preoperative state of the heart, and optimization of myocardial preservation during the procedure, are widely accepted as key factors determining the outcome. Clinicians and pathologists alike should be aware of the complexity of the issue when confronted with pathology afflicting prosthetic valves.

Valvar dysfunction

Dysfunction can be due to a variety of causes. In the early days, variance in the size of the ball due to absorption of lipids was a serious problem. The ball turned yellow and became pliable. Fragmentation would occur (Fig. 13.66) with peripheral emboli-zation of fragments or, occasionally, of the ball itself (Fig. 13.67). The incidence of these complications has drastically fallen with improvements in the manufacturing process of the occluders and poppets. Local problems, nonetheless, such as calcific deposits at the base of the valve or formation of rings of fibrous tissue (Fig. 13.68) still pose a problem and, on occasion, cause postoperative prosthetic valvar dysfunction.

Ventricular geometry plays an important role, particularly since the indications for replacement of a valve are no longer dependent upon age. The geometry of the left ventricle, particularly the shape of its outlet, changes with age. Indeed, important moulding occurs within the outflow tract. A subaortic septal bulge is almost invariably present in the elderly person (Fig. 13.69). In addition, the angle between the planes of the orifices of the mitral and aortic valves is less obtuse than in the young. These features together create a setting in which the orifice of the mitral valve tends to face the ventricular septum rather than the apex. This alteration may jeopardize the success of valvar replacement. Use of caged-ball prostheses in the mitral position

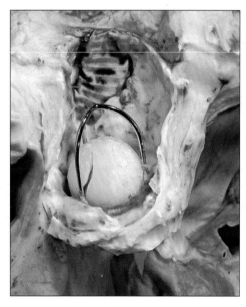

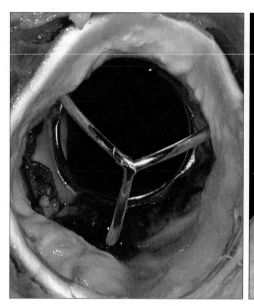

Fig. 13.66 Surgically inserted ball valve. The fragmented ball is yellow because of infiltration of lipids.

Fig. 13.67 Embolism from a caged-ball valve prosthesis: (left) empty cage; (right) ball lodged in abdominal aorta at the iliac bifurcation.

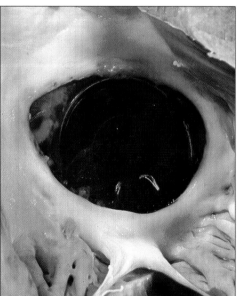

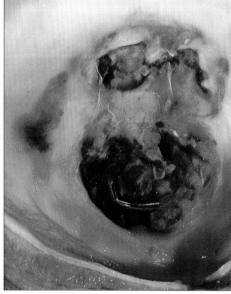

Fig. 13.68 Valvar dysfunction: (left) fibrous ring underneath disc hampering its proper function; (right) atrial aspect of the same prosthetic valve covered by organized thrombus.

has long been known to involve the risk of obstruction to the outflow tract (Fig. 13.70), while septal friction can lead to endocardial fibrosis and, occasionally, septal laceration. The alterations in geometry may also affect the use of other types of artificial valves (Fig. 13.71). Even disc valves may show dysfunction because of an intimate relation between the disc and septum (Fig. 13.72). Prosthetic valvar dysfunction may then trigger the onset of thrombosis, particularly when the dysfunctioning valve is in mitral position (Fig. 13.73). Eventually, the valve may become virtually immobilized by organized thrombus covering its atrial aspect (Fig. 13.68, right). Thrombosis of a prosthetic valve, however, can also occur as a late phenomenon in the agonal state, and is not necessarily related to the principal cause of cardiac deterioration. It is important, therefore, to distinguish these processes.

The main concern regarding the use of bioprostheses is their durability. Dysfunction due to calcification of the leaflets is well documented. This phenomenon is particularly likely to occur in young patients. Biochemical changes of collagen, in part induced by the pretreatment with glutaraldehyde together with deposition of thrombi, play a major role in the pathogenesis of calcification. The precise mechanisms, however, remain controversial.

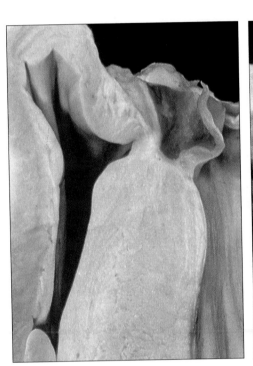

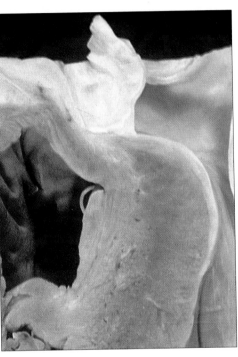

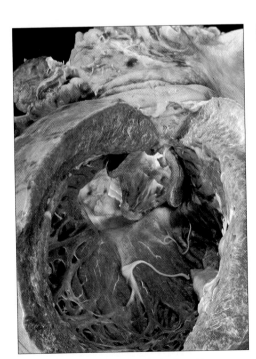

Fig. 13.69 The outflow tract from the left ventricle is almost straight in the young (left) but shows subvalvar bulging in the elderly (right).

Fig. 13.70 Caged-ball prostheses in both aortic and mitral positions. The mitral prosthesis obstructs the outlet from the left ventricle.

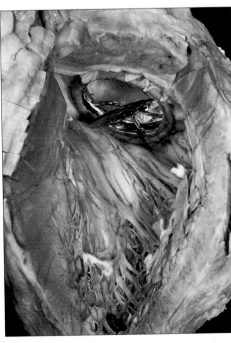

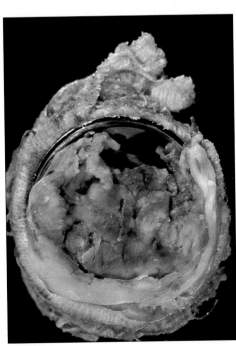

Fig. 13.71 Bioprosthesis in mitral position obstructing the outlet from the left ventricle.

Fig. 13.72 Disc valve in mitral position showing intimate contact between the disc and the ventricular septum leading to valvar dysfunction.

Fig. 13.73 Surgically excised prosthetic mitral valve almost completely covered by thrombus.

Injury and laceration

In the early period of closed commissurotomy for rheumatic stenosis of the mitral valve, the aortic or mural leaflets were sometimes split instead of the commissure (Fig. 13.74). Even when properly executed, insufficiency following commissurotomy was a problem. Restenosis was largely determined by the pre-existent valvar pathology. These complications have subsided since the introduction of open heart procedures.

Insertion of a prosthetic valve may induce myocardial laceration. Injuries to the atrioventricular junction are more likely in hearts with calcifications that extend into the myocardium or, in cases of pathology involving the aortic or mitral valve, onto its neighbouring valve. Removal of excess tissue to permit implantation of the prosthesis may lead to separation of the left atrium from the left ventricle, or of the aortic root from the base of the heart. Hence, false aneurysms develop at these sites. The close relation between the aortic valve and the atrioventricular conduction tissues is well recognized, and heart block following surgery on the aortic valve is extremely rare. Transverse ventricular disruption is an important, though often concealed, complication (Fig. 13.75). Hearts with chronic rheumatic disease of the mitral valve are prone to this form of injury. Direct surgical trauma is unlikely. The pathogenetic mechanism promoted is that of disruption of an important functional longitudinal binder by detachment of the papillary muscles from the mitral valve, thus permitting stretch damage to the myocardium.

A particular type of injury is the occurrence of perioperative myocardial infarction. Improved techniques for myocardial preservation have minimized this risk. Direct injury to coronary arteries can occur, but this complication is extremely rare. The circumflex artery is especially at risk when replacing a diseased mitral valve with extensive calcification of the atrioventricular junction (Fig. 13.76).

Stenosis of a prosthetic valve in the aortic position is an important cause of postoperative low cardiac output (Fig. 13.77) when the diameter of the aortic root is too small for the prosthesis inserted. Undue stretch of the aortic root, moreover, transforms the orifices of the coronary arteries into narrowed slit-like structures (Fig. 13.78). Myocardial perfusion is then further jeopardized. Since preoperative assessment of the size of the aortic root may prevent this complication, and with improving experience in handling these conditions at surgery, this form of pathology is becoming less significant. In some patients, nonetheless, primarily those with prosthetic valves placed in both aortic and mitral position, the postoperative period may be complicated by progressive pump failure of the left ventricle which then leads to death. No apparent cause can be demonstrated at autopsy. It may well be that a similar, but more complex, situation is occurring in these cases. It should not be forgotten that, during the period of disease, the heart has adjusted to the gradually progressive changes in valvar pathology. The whole scene is abruptly changed when the surgeon creates unobstructed blood flow through the orifices. An unstable equilibrium built up over the years suddenly collapses, and the myocardium is unable to cope with the new situation at such short notice.

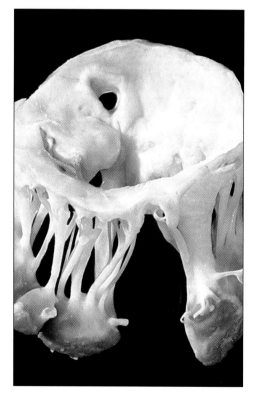

Fig. 13.74 Surgically resected rheumatic mitral valve showing a split in the aortic leaflet due to false route from previous commissurotomy.

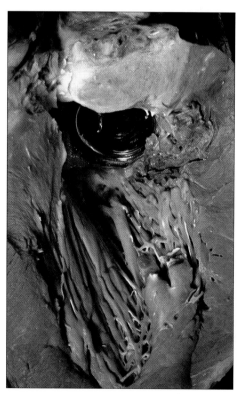

Fig. 13.75 Transverse ventricular laceration following replacement of the mitral valve.

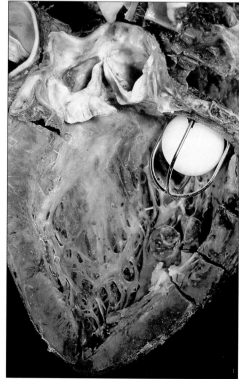

Fig. 13.76 Inferior and lateral infarction of the left ventricle produced by injury to the circumflex artery during replacement of the mitral valve.

Dehiscence of valves

Dehiscence of prosthetic valves, leading to a so-called paravalvar leak, may be an early complication. It usually results from faulty surgical technique. Small openings are mostly due to retraction of tissues from the sewing ring (Fig. 13.79). A large dehiscence almost always occurs because stitches pull apart. Pre-existent abnormalities, such as infarction or secondary infection, play an important role. In time, the edges of the paravalvar leak become smooth and lined by thickened endocardium. An endocardial jet lesion may develop secondary to the localized regurgitant flow (Fig. 13.80). Although small openings are usually considered of little clinical relevance, it is our experience that, on occasion, a small dehiscence will have important haemodynamic consequences. Thus, an annuloplasty of the tricuspid valve became forcefully disrupted when a small paravalvar leak along a prosthesis inserted in mitral position, sought but not found at operation, was left unclosed.

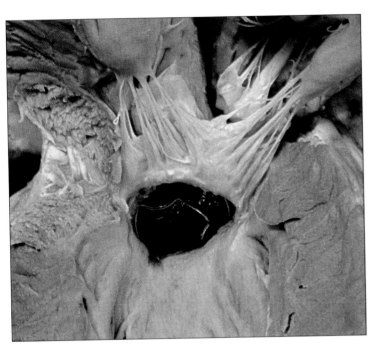

Fig. 13.77 Prosthetic valvar stenosis: a disc valve in aortic position is in excess of the diameter of the orifice.

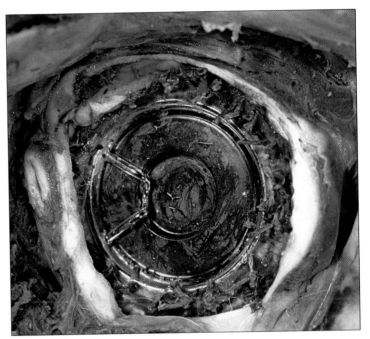

Fig. 13.78 Disproportionate prosthetic valve in aortic position leading to stretching of aortic root and slit-like transformation of the orifices of the coronary arteries.

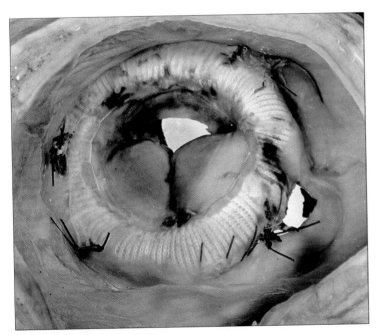

Fig. 13.79 Paravalvar leak due to dehiscence of the valvar ring.

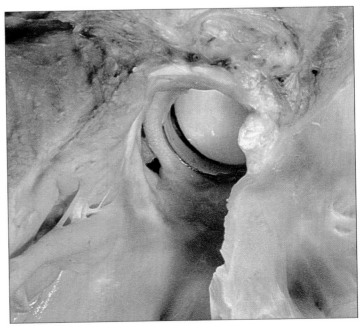

Fig. 13.80 Paravalvar leak along a mechanical valve inserted in aortic position showing an endocardial jet lesion on ventricular septum.

Infection of prosthetic valves

Any prosthetic valve is liable to endocarditis. The coating of the valve ring and sutures by platelets and fibrin serve as niduses for infection. Endocarditis of porcine xenografts almost always involves the leaflets and, most likely, develops from within the deposits of fibrin overlying their surfaces.

Hence, infection in mechanical prostheses usually leads to detachment (Fig. 13.81) and formation of abscesses in the junction, whereas disruption of leaflets is the dominating feature of infection of a bioprosthesis (Fig. 13.82).

As with infective endocarditis in general (see above), almost any organism is capable of producing prosthetic endocarditis. The infection is basically destructive in nature. The infected area is usually covered by thrombi (Fig. 13.83) which often leads to impaired function of the valve and septic thromboembolization. Mycotic aneurysms of the ascending aorta may occur, either at the site of the aortic incision or due to mechanical trauma produced by the struts of the prosthesis (Fig. 13.84). Prophylactic treatment with antibiotics is advisable in all patients who have had surgery on cardiac valves, irrespective of the type of valve inserted, whenever the patient subsequently undergoes a procedure likely to produce bacteraemia.

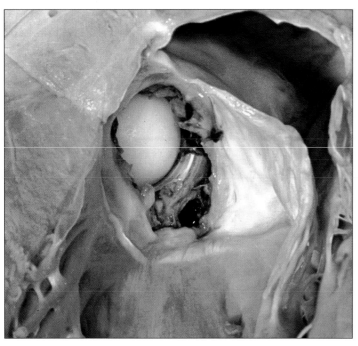

Fig. 13.81 Infection of a mechanical valve inserted in aortic position leading to dehiscence of the valve.

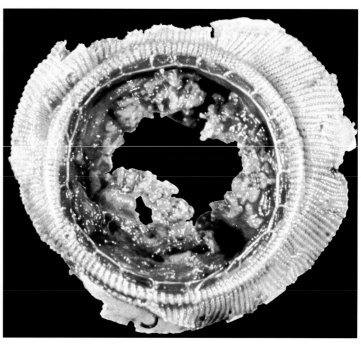

Fig. 13.82 Infective endocarditis of a Hancock bioprosthesis with disruption of the valvar tissue. By courtesy of Prof G. Thiene.

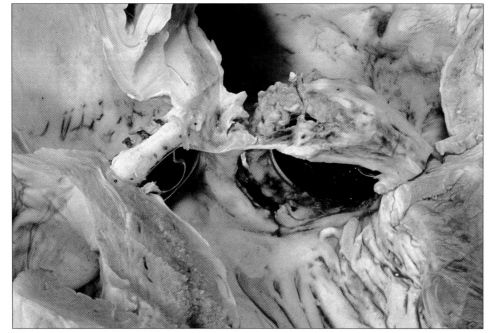

Fig. 13.83 Infection of disc valve in mitral position leading to dehiscence at the ring and excessive thrombosis covering the site of infection. Note the disc valve in aortic position.

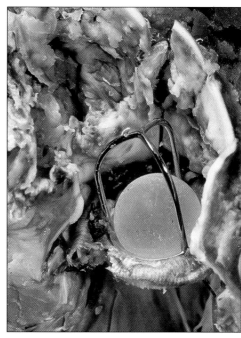

Fig. 13.84 Late infection of the ascending aorta following replacement of the aortic valve.

15   THE AGEING HEART

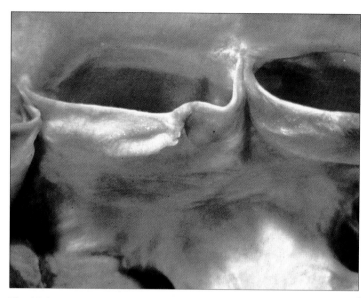

Fig. 15.1   Aortic valve of an elderly person. The line of closure is eccentrically accentuated. The leaflets are thickened due to fibrosis. Note yellowish plaques on the aortic leaflet of the mitral valve.

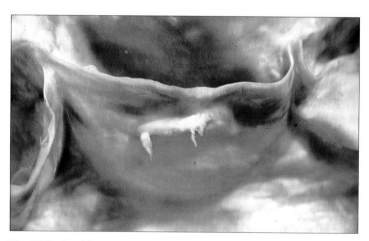

Fig. 15.2   Lambl's excrescences on the aortic valve.

In the Western world, increasing longevity has led to a corresponding waxing interest in geriatric medicine. In the heart, the most prominent ageing changes relate to the supportive tissues, that is, the fibrous skeleton and the valves.

There are many disease processes which increase in incidence with age, such as atherosclerosis, myocardial hypertrophy, interstitial myocardial fibrosis on the basis of impaired myocardial perfusion, and so-called senile cardiac amyloidosis. None of these conditions, however, can be considered an ageing process in the strict sense.

General aspects

The cardiac valves are thin and transparent at birth. With age, the atrial aspect of the atrioventricular valves and the ventricular surface of the arterial valves thicken because of fibrosis. In addition, the line of closure becomes accentuated (Fig. 15.1) with the development of so-called Lambl's excrescences (Fig. 15.2). These papillary outgrowths, composed of a fibrous core with scattered concentrically-arranged elastic fibres, are particularly prominent on the aortic and mitral valves. The tricuspid (Fig. 15.3) and the pulmonary valves are only rarely involved. These 'natural' changes have long been considered of no clinical relevance. They could, however, play a role in serving as nidi for infective endocarditis (see Section 5), and may be further aggravated by additional pathologic conditions, such as raised pressures and regurgitant flow. The development of almost tumour-like papillary lesions may occasionally happen (Fig. 15.4) and their distinction from papillary fibroelastoma (see Chapter 16) may then become almost impossible. It is extremely difficult, if not impossible, to indicate precisely, in any given individual, where the natural process of physiological ageing ends and pathology begins.

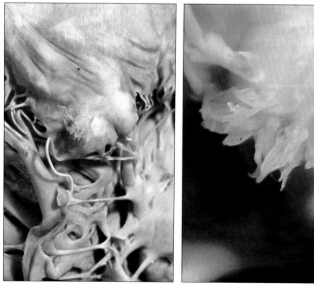

Fig. 15.3   Lambl's excrescences on the tricuspid valve: (left) general view; (right) detail.

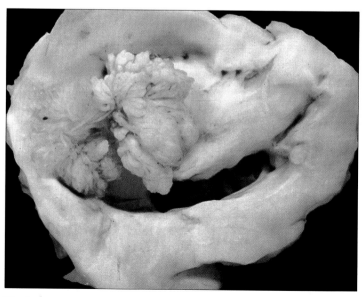

Fig. 15.4   Tumour-like papillary lesion on atrial aspect of aortic leaflet of surgically excised rheumatic mitral valve.

The aortic valve

In the elderly, valve fibrosis is often accompanied by a separation of leaflets from the aortic root along the base of their semilunar attachments. Degenerative changes occur in the supportive tissues and secondary dystrophic calcifications ensue (Fig. 15.5). This process results in spotty calcifications which are seen mainly within the sinuses, at the base and on the aortic aspect of the leaflets. The valve so affected is often described as having 'aortic valve sclerosis'. This usually has little haemodynamic consequences other than producing the harsh systolic ejection murmur which is often audible in older people. The degenerative process that causes this is generally considered to be the consequence of wear and tear and the changes are, in fact, similar to those seen in degenerative aortic valvar stenosis (see Section 5), albeit in a mitigated form. From a pathogenetic viewpoint, however, the two processes can be considered as extremes in a spectrum of ageing that affects the aortic valve and, eventually, may cause stenosis (Fig. 15.6).

The mitral valve

The mitral valve may similarly exhibit degenerative changes. These changes result in valvar fibrosis with accentuation of the line of closure (see above), but, in addition, become prominent at the 'hinge' with the ventricular wall, and at sites of insertion of tendinous cords. Lipid accumulation, often grossly visible (Fig. 15.7), is an almost constant finding at these sites in adults over 40 years of age. Histologically, moreover, marked alterations are found in the staining characteristics of the collagen (Fig. 15.8), indicating a degenerative process. This may render the tissues susceptible to calcium deposition, and the process of 'wear and tear' in the mitral valve may progress, eventually, to a stage known as calcified mitral ring. The latter condition, particularly when clinically relevant, has a distinct preference for females, although the mechanisms which underlie this increased susceptibility remain unclear.

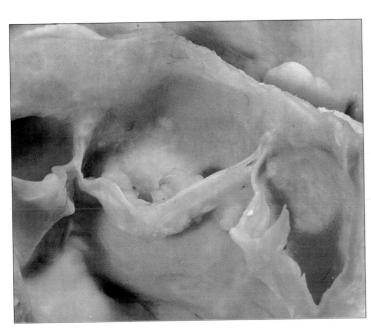

Fig. 15.5 Spotty calcifications inside the leaflets of the aortic valve cusps is a typical change in the elderly.

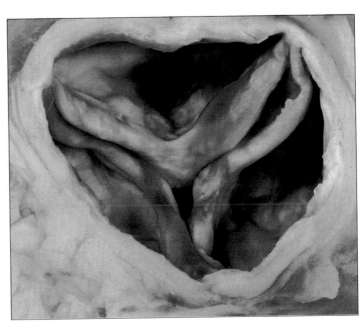

Fig. 15.6 Stenosis of the aortic valve secondary to advanced ageing changes. Note absence of commissural fusion.

Fig. 15.7 Ventricular aspect of the mitral valve at site of insertion into ventricular wall. Note spotty lipid accumulations.

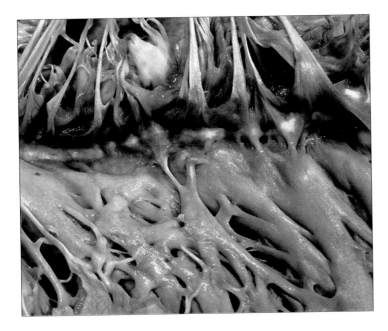

Calcification of the mitral ring in its classical form presents as a horseshoe-shaped ridge (Fig. 15.9) on the ventricular surface of the mitral valve. The calcific deposits are localized in the angle between the leaflets and the ventricular wall, and usually extend onto the valve leaflet to incorporate cordal attachments. The lesion may be confined to the middle part of the mural leaflet (Fig. 15.10) or it may extend in an almost circular fashion (Fig. 15.11). Massive calcification can occur, immobilizing the greater part of the valve leaflet (Fig. 15.12). Mitral insufficiency is the usual clinical feature under these circumstances. The calcific deposits may also extend into the myocardium of the left ventricular free wall (Fig. 15.13), and the calcified ring can show central softening, rather like a caseous abscess. It probably reflects the structural alteration in the composition of collagen, basic to the anomaly, but without much calcium deposited as yet.

Thrombosis can occur beneath the leaflets of the mitral valve, in a position which corresponds to the calcified ring (Fig. 15.14). Thrombotic deposits may eventually organize and calcify, but subvalvar thrombosis is no longer considered to be the underlying pathogenetic mechanism in the appearance of mitral calcification. The combined occurrence of calcific aortic disease and calcified mitral ring is a particularly common finding in the elderly (Fig. 15.15).

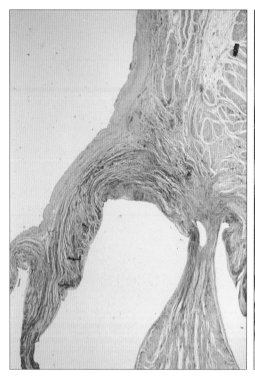

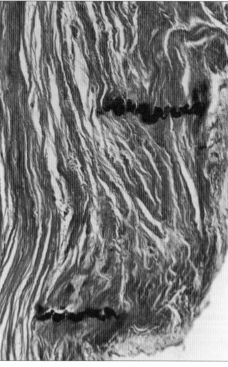

Fig. 15.8 Histological appearance of an ageing mitral valve. The left hand panel shows the valve at the atrioventricular junction. At the base of the valve leaflet, close to the insertion of a cord, irregular cross bands appear stained intensely red, as a sign of collagen degeneration. The right hand panel shows the area in more detail.

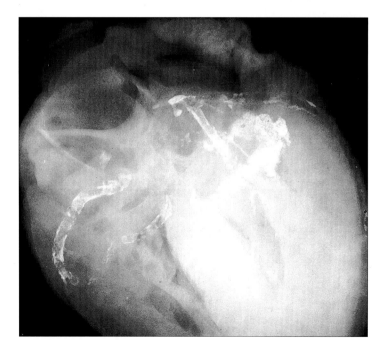

Fig. 15.9 Post-mortem radiograph showing horseshoe-shaped calcification in the mitral valve. The coronary arteries also exhibit marked calcifications of their walls.

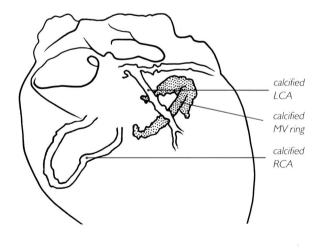

calcified LCA

calcified MV ring

calcified RCA

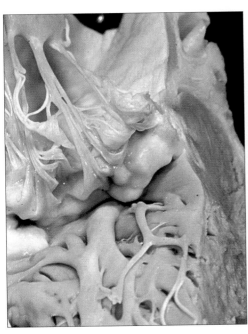

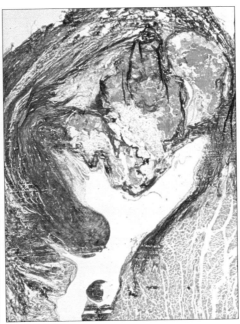

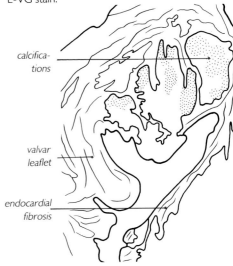

Fig. 15.10 Calcified mitral ring: (left) calcific deposits beneath the mural leaflet of the valve; (right) histology showing calcified mass in base of leaflet; note endocardial fibrosis as friction lesion. E-VG stain.

calcifica-
tions

valvar
leaflet

endocardial
fibrosis

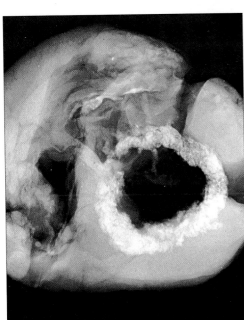

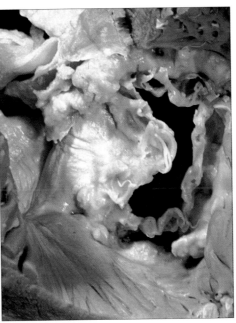

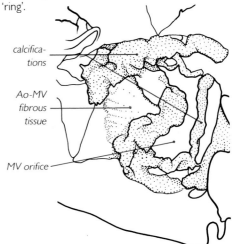

Fig. 15.11 Calcified mitral ring: (left) post-mortem radiograph, craniocaudal view, showing ring-like calcification of the valvar orifice; (right) ventricular aspect exhibiting subvalvar calcifications extending onto fibrous tissue, thus completing the 'ring'.

calcifica-
tions

Ao-MV
fibrous
tissue

MV orifice

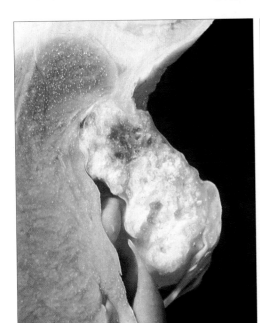

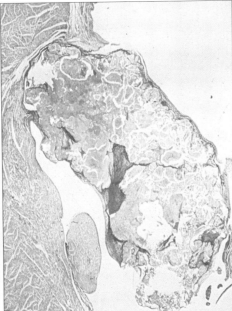

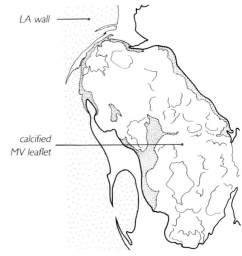

Fig. 15.12 Calcified mitral ring: (left) extensive calcification of the leaflet; only the most distal part of the leaflet is pliable; (right) histology reveals massive involvement of leaflet and its cordal attachments. E-VG stain.

LA wall

calcified
MV leaflet

Right heart valves

Ageing changes in the right heart are less outspoken than the left-sided changes, although the large anterosuperior leaflet of the tricuspid valve almost always shows fibrous thickening (Fig. 15.16). In elderly patients with pulmonary disease and right ventricular hypertrophy, the atrial surface of the leaflets may be highly irregular, with surface depositions of fibrin, resembling ulceration. The pulmonary valve shows similar fibrosis, particularly in cases with sustained pulmonary hypertension, irrespective of its cause.

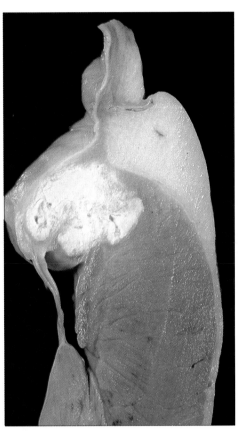

Fig. 15.13 Calcified mitral ring extending into myocardium. The central part is soft, exhibiting a superficial resemblance to caseous necrosis.

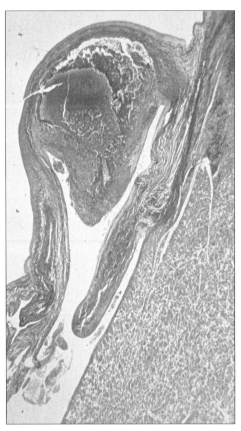

Fig. 15.14 Partially organized subvalvar thrombosis. E-VG stain.

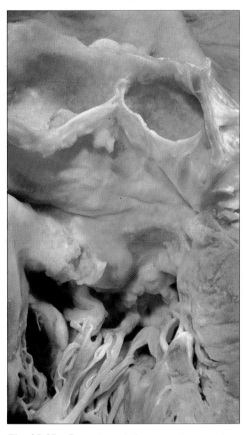

Fig. 15.15 Extensive calcific ageing changes of the apparatus of both aortic and mitral valves. Calcific deposits extend onto the ventricular septum.

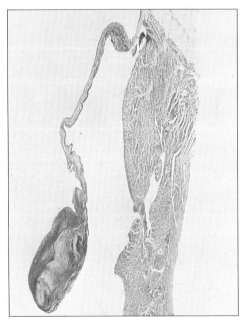

Fig. 15.16 Histology of leaflet of the tricuspid valve with marked fibrosis on atrial aspect. E-VG stain.

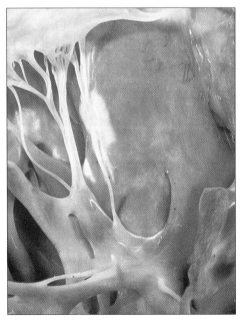

Fig. 15.17 Friction lesions of cords: fibrous lesion on right ventricular aspect of septum encapsulating cord.

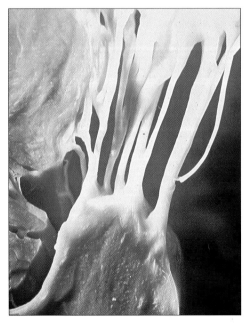

Fig. 15.18 Fibrous encasement of cords of the mitral valve.

Endocardium

Endocardial thickening frequently occurs in relation to tendinous cords. These friction, or rub, lesions are particularly prominent in hearts with ventricular hypertrophy. Septal lesions are commonly seen in association with right ventricular hypertrophy (Fig. 15.17), whereas, with left ventricular hypertrophy, lesions are often encountered in the posterobasal aspect (Fig. 15.18). These lesions may progress from small imprints of overlying cords to large fibrous encapsulations of one or several cords. The larger examples may contribute to impaired function of the valve and, occasionally, form the nidus for mural endocarditis. The incidence of endocardial friction and rub lesions increases with age, but their appearance is enhanced by other circumstances. From that point of view, therefore, these changes should not be considered ageing changes in the strict sense.

The cardiac skeleton and conduction

The process of 'wear and tear' of the cardiac skeleton probably underlies the gradual separation of the aortic root from the ventricular septum in the elderly. This contributes to the so-called sigmoid septum and the altered geometry of the left ventricular outflow tract (see also Section 5).

Calcification of the central fibrous body can also occur (Fig. 15.19, left), whereby the calcified mass may extend onto the ventricular septum and impinge on the atrioventricular bundle and bundle branches, thus producing heart block (Fig. 15.19, right). The calcific mass in these instances represents the end-stage of a process of 'wear and tear' of the central fibrous body. This is relevant since the conduction tissues have to pass through the fibrous skeleton in order to descend onto the ventricular myocardium (see also Chapter 1). Consequently, the disintegration of the cardiac skeleton may lead to attenuation and fibrosis of the conduction fibres. This degenerative process probably underlies the common finding of proximal atrioventricular dissociation, known as Lev's disease, in elderly patients. The fibrocalcific nature of this disease should be distinguished from idiopathic bundle branch fibrosis, known as Lenègre's disease, which affects the more peripheral parts of the bundle branch system.

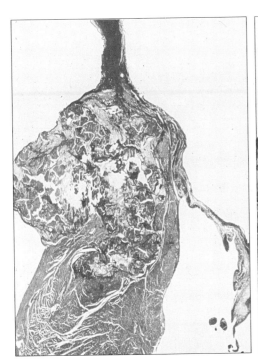
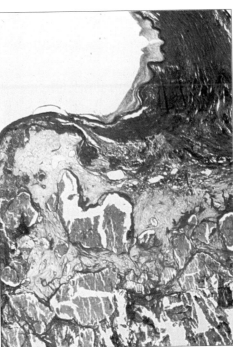

Fig. 15.19 Histological section showing extensive septal calcifications as part of age-related pathology: (left) general view; (right) detail. The left bundle is entrapped by massive calcifications. E-VG stain.

membranous septum

area of calcifications

MV

TV

ventricular septum

membranous septum

LBB

calcifications in septum

Insertion of pacemakers

In cases of heart block, the insertion of pacemakers may intro-
duce other forms of pathology. They carry a particular risk
of producing endocardial laceration and of providing nests for
thrombosis and infection. The incidence of these complications
is directly related to the amount of time a catheter is in place.
Thrombosis rapidly develops as heat around the catheter
and is particularly likely to develop at sites of endocardial
laceration. The thrombotic event may give rise to further
complications, such as inlet obstruction or thromboembolism.
Infection is a most serious complication, albeit rare.
When it does occur, the removal of the pacemaker is usually
necessary for complete recovery, regardless of whether the lead
is endocardial or pericardial.

In time, catheters can become partly encapsulated by fibrous
tissue. These fibrous sheaths favour sites of mural contact and
electrode catheters left in place for a long time may become
encased within the right atrium, usually near the entrance of
the superior caval vein. Such encasement also occurs at
the site of contact with the tricuspid valve and within
the right ventricle, usually near the apex where the catheter
tip is lodged between trabeculations. However, Tricuspid
insufficiency is relatively uncommon, despite fibrous encasement
and secondary reactive changes. In addition, proper pacemaker
function is rarely interfered with by the development of fibrous
tissue at the electrode tip, although the changes which are evoked
remain as possible sites for infective endocarditis.